What Others Ar

INTUITIVE HEALTH

"Alli accounts for herself very admirably, using her own real, honest, genuine and authentic voice. She talks to you through the text as if you were in the living room discussing important aspects of your life, gently coaxing you to think deeply about what is going on, and suggesting some ways you might approach matters in a very positive way. With the addition of questionnaires the book truly becomes an owner's manual for life and life improvement. I recommend you grab a copy and then you'll know too that Alli is sincere in her desire for you to put her knowledge to work for yourself. Consider it an easy read, with homework, and you'll be on your way to transforming yourself inside and out."

Reed Davis
Founder, Functional Diagnostic Nutrition® Program

"Alli Gardner is clearing the air about nutrition. Everyone wants out of the Standard American Diet, but no one wants another diet cult or theory. Alli clears the air, with common sense, and reassurance. What she's written here will have her readers' feet planted firmly on the ground, guided to a fearless way of making choices about food! A must read for everyone looking for the truth in health and nutrition."

Robyn Openshaw
GreenSmoothieGirl.com and GSGLife.com

"Alli's book presents a plan that allows individuals to make substantive and positive changes to their lives without feeling rushed or stressed. By acknowledging that not one size fits all Alli gives the reader tools to make the positive changes most important to them and to make those changes last. If you've ever wondered what your first step should be in a journey towards health, this is a place to start."

Matthew Burnett, ND
Utah Natural Medicine

"Alli Gardner's book allows you to go deeper into understanding your beliefs about health, food, body and weight so that you can create a life lasting transformation versus a quick fix. If you're a busy woman struggling with weight, body and food; this is a must read. You'll be able to relate to Alli's real life journey of balancing it all- family, health and fitness and finding freedom through intuitive eating! Enjoy!"

Amanda Moxley CHHC, CSW
The Healthy Wealthy Biz Mentor

INTUITIVE HEALTH

Transform Yourself
From The Inside Out

Alli Gardner

Kelley,
Enjoy your journey!
In health & happiness,

INTUITIVE HEALTH
Transform Yourself From The Inside Out
by Alli Gardner

A Message to the Reader

The information provided in this book is designed to provide helpful information on the subjects discussed. This book is not meant to be used, nor should it be used, to diagnose or treat any medical condition. For diagnosis or treatment of any medical problem, consult your own physician. The author is not responsible for any specific health or allergy needs that may require medical supervision and is not liable for any damages or negative consequences from any treatment, action, application or preparation, to any person reading or following the information in this book. References are provided for informational purposes only and do not constitute endorsement of any websites or other sources. Readers should be aware that the websites listed in this book may change.

CONTENTS

WHAT IS INTUITIVE HEALTH?

WHY DO YOU WANT TO IMPROVE YOUR HEALTH?

WHAT SHOULD I CHANGE AND
WHAT DO I WANT TO ACHIEVE?

HOW DO I ACTUALLY MAKE CHANGES
IN MY HABITS AND HEALTH?

KNOWLEDGE IS POWER

ENJOY YOUR LIFE

APPENDIX

Section I

What Is Intuitive Health?

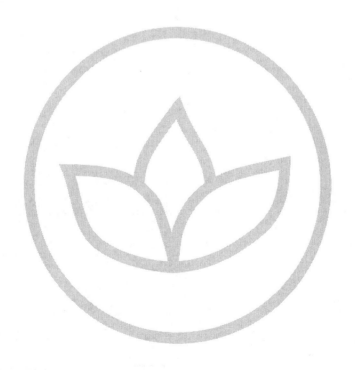

Health Is a Journey

A man with his health has many dreams.
A man without his health has but one.

Anonymous

In this era of technology, information is abundant. Have a question? Google it. Have a health concern? Turn to the Internet or seek the advice of a doctor or friend. You may receive an answer that doesn't make sense to you. You follow the recommendations anyway but to no avail. You continue looking and questioning.

You search Amazon.com for books on weight loss and 93,804 possibilities come up. Then you try diet books and the number increases to 99,471. Do they work? Of course, they work for the right people at the right time in their life. Each author believes in what he/she is writing. It worked for the author. Do you continue your quest or do you quit in frustration?

You want to be healthy. But what does it mean to be healthy?

May I suggest that being healthy is not a destination. It is a journey. Many of you have a goal of being healthy, but do you really know what you are trying to achieve? Whose standards of health are you trying to achieve? By health, are you merely trying to not be sick, to avoid illness, cancer, heart disease, and diabetes? Do you intend to lead a life full of energy and happiness, and enjoy your friends and loved ones? In your pursuit of health are you focused on a particular weight? Perhaps you want a certain look in order to "fit in." We all possess a personal definition of health. Thus, we should all have a unique approach to achieving health - an approach that is unique to us.

The Institute of Integrative Nutrition (IIN), where I studied nutrition, provides information and training on hundreds of dietary theories. The creator of each theory is passionately convinced that theirs is the path to health. I found myself believing that what they were teaching was the way to go. I experimented a lot during that year. I ate a more raw based diet. I eliminated dairy. I practiced a gluten free diet. I ate more animal protein. What I lost was focus. What I gained was frustration. I hungered to find the easy button: tell me what to eat, how much to eat, and when to eat it. Eventually I accepted what I knew was truth but had chosen to ignore: there is no easy button. When it comes to health and nutrition, we are all unique. What works for me may or may not work for you entirely. Nutrition is not black and white. It is not as easy as eat this and never eat that. You are human and you will make mistakes. Once you give yourself permission to experiment and make mistakes, you will begin to correlate your actions with your feelings and your health. You will learn what works best for you.

Life is dynamic. Health is dynamic. You are getting older every second that passes. Your cells that make up your entire matter are constantly regenerating. In the course of one year, every cell in your body has regenerated. That means it is never too late to start over and do better. You can undo the mistakes you made and move forward. It's never too late to change your lifestyle and habits. But you have to be willing to make the first move. You have to step out of your comfort zone and be vulnerable. You have to be willing to make mistakes and to ask questions. You have to be willing to do what is best for you. Change is both uncomfortable and exhilarating. Once you are ready to change your life and your health, anything is possible.

My intention with this book is to guide you to discover your own path to health and happiness. Health is not just about what you eat, how much you weigh, or how often you exercise. Health is about living the life of your dreams. It is having the balance of mind, body, and soul that allows you to achieve your goals and to be who you want to be. It is about listening to your inner voice. Health is about having the confidence to follow your gut and make the decisions that are best for you. Only you know what's best for you. You are the one who has your best interest at heart.

Intuitive Health

This is a new era of health and medicine. Studies abound that discuss the relationship between nutrition and health. Food is fundamental to our well-being. According to the Center for Disease Control, in 2012 more than one third of Americans, adults and children, were considered overweight or obese. Childhood obesity is the number one health concern among parents. Former Surgeon General Richard Carmona said, "Because of the increasing rates of obesity, unhealthy eating habits, and physical inactivity, we may see the first generation that will be less healthy and have a shorter life expectancy than their parents." Now is the time to make changes, not only in the foods we eat and our activity levels, but also in our thoughts and habits around food. There is no quick fix. Everyone wants the easy answer: the magic pill to lose 30 pounds in 30 days without changing diet and without exercise; a seven-minute exercise program; a special diet to improve health. We spend money and become discouraged when the easy way to lose weight doesn't work, or it only works temporarily.

Being healthy, through nutrition and exercise, is not difficult. What is challenging is creating the habits that foster great health. Improving your health is all about consistency. Start with adding one new habit at a time. With persistence, that habit will become automatic, or part of your daily routine. You then add another habit and another until you are consistently and subconsciously making decisions that will better your health. This book does not come with an easy button to activate. I'm not going to tell you what to eat or what to do for exercise. I'm not going to list "superfoods" that will guarantee your health for years to come.

My intention is to enlighten you on a new way of viewing your health. I want to give you the tools and the knowledge so you can make the decisions to improve you health on your own. Move slowly and implement one new health habit at a time. Each habit will build upon the previous one. This will establish your foundation.

Intuitive health means listening to your body and using your intuition to guide your decisions. You slow down and learn to listen to what your mind, body, and soul are telling you. You connect your behaviors with how you feel. You make changes to improve your life. Why do some people make this seem so easy, while others struggle to follow their intuition? Is intuition something you either have or your don't? Is intuition something that can be taught?

We all have intuition. You have to train yourself to listen. It is easy to get caught up in the world around you and start following a path that is not true to your life purpose and your values. You listen to other voices around you - other people telling you what to do. You do what others think you should do rather than doing what you believe and know is best for you. You get caught up in making the right decision or doing the right things. In life, there is no 'right' answer. Every decision you make is taking you closer to your end goal. It may not be a straight course but when you go with your feelings and your end goal in mind, every decision you make has a purpose. Every decision you have made has brought you to the point you are at today. If you would like to be at a different point, you have complete control to make decisions to reach that point.

As I look back on my life, my greatest regrets or poorest decisions were made because I didn't follow my gut. I made decisions based on what others (society, friends, etc.) were telling me to do, not what I knew I was supposed to do. I've made huge decisions quickly in the past few years with confidence because I knew I was following my intuition and it would all work out. I haven't been let down. I'm not saying that my life has turned out exactly as I had planned, I'm not a fortuneteller, but my life is turning out great.

I once said, "I must have good luck, things always seem to go my way and work out." A friend replied, "That's not good luck, it's that you always adapt and make the most of the life that is in front of you."

We are too critical of ourselves. We are overcome with fear of making a mistake so we do nothing. We change nothing. In the grand scheme of things, are there really right and wrong decisions? Even apparent wrong decisions turn out to be valuable learning experiences that guide and shape us into who we are. When we face a big decision, we can experience paralysis of analysis. We analyze and analyze and never make a decision. Our life stagnates. We never move forward. Life without change leads to an unfulfilled existence. Change can be difficult but it fosters growth. Wouldn't it be nice to learn to follow your heart and make decisions with confidence knowing that it will all work out because you are doing what you are supposed to be doing? What a great world that would be! Decisions would be made with a grand purpose rather than making decisions based on what appears right, or what others tell you, or what you think you are supposed to do.

You ask others for their opinion because you lack the confidence to follow your intuition. You want them to validate your thoughts. When they offer a different perspective, you have so much information it becomes impossible to make a decision and move forward. You become confused. You lose your ability to listen to your own intuition, the inner voice that guides us in the right direction. Making decisions can be overwhelming. Learning to trust your intuition is a process.

Watch a child use a computer. They are fearless. They keep trying until they get it right. They don't worry about the consequences. They just push buttons until they get the response they are looking for. What if you were fearless when it came to making decisions about your health? It would alter your entire perception as well as your actions. . The media telling you to eat this and don't eat that, exercise this way and not like that, do yoga, meditate this way bombard you. Then a new study appears that contradicts everything. You either follow the latest fads with the intention of finding something that works, or you do nothing for fear of not doing the right thing. I offer a different approach.

What if every decision you made was based on your inner voice? You make mistakes but learn from them. You stay positive knowing that you're doing the best you can and continue to move toward your destination. You cut yourself some slack and dig deep into your subconscious to figure what's really going on. Don't worry about what the right answer is or what the right decision is, just do the best you can and move forward.

As you make decisions, keep your values and conscience in mind. If you make your own decisions by following your intuition then you cannot go wrong. You inherently know what is best for you. When you make decisions based on outsiders' suggestions, you frequently go astray from your core values and beliefs. You live a life that is out of alignment with your true essence.

Intuition is the ability to know that something is true without having objective data to support your beliefs. It is a feeling that you know something to be true. Listening to your intuition and letting it guide you takes practice. It is a learned skill to have the faith and confidence to follow your intuition. By listening to your body, you make decisions that are best for you. You listen to what your body craves and give your body what it needs to flourish. This allows you to have energy and health, in order to live the life of your dreams.

As creatures of habit, we have a tendency to go through life on autopilot. We make decisions regarding our health and the foods we eat without thinking. We eat foods that we have always eaten. It is difficult to break these habits that are engrained in our subconscious. When it comes to making decisions regarding our health, we need to question these decisions. Are you making your daily decisions out of habit, or because you read it somewhere, or because you are listening to your intuition and choosing what's best for you and your health that day? When you get caught up in this crazy world of information, you stop making decisions based on your own feelings and emotions. You forget to listen to what is really best for you. Slow down, and become more mindful of the decisions you make each day. Work to create a habit of health.

When you approach any new journey or challenge in life, you must ask three fundamental questions.

- ❧ Why?
- ❧ What?
- ❧ How?

Why?

Why are you ready for change? Why do you want to be healthy? Understanding and embracing your why is paramount in your success. When you see the big picture and have a deep understanding of the importance, you will be better able to stay on track when challenges and temptations arise.

What?

What changes are you going to make? What is your vision? Once you understand what you want, you will manifest the changes in your life.

How?

How will you make these changes and implement each step to figure out what works best for you? I will guide you to add one new health habit at a time. You will discover your path and take ownership of your health.

In addition to the three critical questions, there is one more element critical for your transformation and that is to live, laugh, learn, and love. Set goals then achieve your goals. Then set new goals and achieve those, too. Your journey doesn't end. You revise the goals and continue.

Live your life to its fullest. Laugh often. Learn all that you can. The more you know, the more empowered you become to make your own decisions. Love deeply.

This book is divided into six sections, with chapters in each section. The chapters in Sections Two, Three, and Four contain a variety of worksheets with questions to help you achieve your transformation. Answer the questions as you go. The worksheets are found in the appendix, in the accompanying workbook, and they can be downloaded from my website at www.alligardner.com/bookbonus. The fifth section, Knowledge Is Power, is divided into chapters so you can skip around to read each chapter in the order that suits you best. I have written two case studies at the end of the book for guidance as well as my personal journey.

It is important that you read through sections two through four and fill in the worksheets in order to build a foundation. This will guide your decisions as you begin to implement new habits. Once you have identified the first habit you will implement, read that chapter in Section Five to get you started. You will build on each chapter as you add new habits.

Section II

Why Do You Want to Improve Your Health?

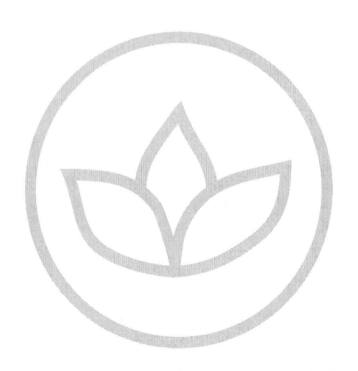

Find Your WHY

The thing about health is that it's not just about one thing. If you want to lose weight, it's not just about changing what you eat. That's a big part of it but that's not the whole story. To be truly healthy and happy you must find balance in your life. You have to look at all aspects of your life to determine what is out of alignment and creating a situation, which has kept you from achieving your goals. First you must understand why you want to make changes and why these changes are important in your life.

You need to identify why you want to achieve your goals. Maybe you would like to lose weight. Maybe you want to feel better and have more energy. Maybe you just don't feel right and aren't happy and want to change. Maybe you are unsatisfied at work or under an enormous amount of stress, which now affects your health. Whatever is the reason, pain, or motivation, you have to ask why - dig deep and ask why? Why do you want to lose weight? Why do you want to feel better and have more energy? Why aren't you happy? Why do you want to improve your health?

At first glance, you can give the easy, superficial, textbook answer, but I want you to look deep inside at the root of it. You also have to create your own definition of health. Answer the following questions to identify your Why. Refer to the handout, "Why Health," in the Intuitive Health Workbook.

What does it mean to be healthy to you?

Do you meet your own definition of health? Why or Why not?

How will you feel when you are healthy?

How will you look when you are healthy?

How will being healthy affect your life?

How will being healthy affect those closest to you?

What do you feel is holding you back from being healthy?

How long have you been working to improve your health?

What has prevented you from improving your health?

Why do you want to improve your health?

Are you ready and willing to do whatever it takes to improve your health?

Identify Who You Are and
Why You Are the Way You Are

My goal for you is that great health becomes a habit. It is not about being perfect. It is about making progress. That means making the best decision you can in each given situation. It is about moving forward, even when you make a poor decision. It is about loving yourself and your journey. The decisions you make are largely shaped by your past: by the way you were raised, the environment you grew up in, the people you were surrounded by. Since you are shaped by your past, let's spend a moment and think about why you are the way you are. Answer the following questions and refer to the handout, "Who Are You?" in the Intuitive Health Workbook.

What was your childhood like? Describe your family and home life.

What did you do for fun? Were you active as a child?

What foods did you eat?

Were your parents or caregivers healthy? Were they active?

How did your parents or caregivers handle stress? Did they exercise, turn to food, drink alcohol or smoke, yell?

Do you see any of these behaviors in your own life? If so, which ones?

How do you handle stress? How does it affect your life?

Does this bring up any behaviors that you would like to change? If so, what are they?

Why do you want to change these behaviors?

How do these behaviors relate to your health?

Whom Does Your Behavior and Health Affect?

As you begin to change your life and create new habits, it is important to realize that you are not the only one affected by your changes. Your success will have a great impact on everyone around you: your significant other, your children, your parents, your co-workers, and your friends, really everyone you come into contact with. As you improve your life, you will change the energy that surrounds you. Your vibration will increase. You are raising the bar. Have you ever had the experience of meeting someone who just draws you in? You may not be able to describe it but you just love their energy and the vibration they give off. You want to spend more time with them because just being near them lifts you up. You have probably had the opposite experience with someone who has a negative vibration; they make you feel negative and down. You may not want to spend much time with them because you can feel them bringing you down. As you change your life and become healthier and happier, your vibration will increase. You will find that your relationships change as your habits and vibration improves. Are you ready for this? Sometimes we are not afraid of failing. Instead we are actually afraid of succeeding.

Our deepest fear is not that we are inadequate. Our deepest fear is that we are powerful beyond measure. It is our light, not our darkness that most frightens us. We ask ourselves, who am I to be brilliant, gorgeous, talented, fabulous?

Actually, who are you not to be?

You are a child of God. Your playing small does not serve the world. There is nothing enlightened about shrinking so that other people won't feel insecure around you. We are all meant to shine, as children do. We were born to manifest the glory of God that is within us. It is not just in some of us; it is in everyone. And as we let our own light shine, we unconsciously give other people permission to do the same. As we are liberated from our own fear, our presence automatically liberates others. – Nelson Mandela

Answer the following questions and refer to the handout, "Fears/Support Worksheet" in the Intuitive Health Workbook.

How will your life improve when you achieve your goals?

Who will be affected by your achievement?

How will you feel if you don't achieve your goals?

How will those closest to you be affected if you don't achieve your goals?

Do you have any fears around achieving your goals?

How will you overcome those fears?

What support do you need to achieve your goals?

Who will support you?

Why will you benefit from this support?

When will you ask for support?

Where will you receive support?

Identify Your Limiting Beliefs

Your own beliefs can hold you back or get in your own way of achieving your goals. Your belief system is a combination of things from your childhood: things you have read or seen, things you have been told, or sometimes things you know from your own experiences. Many of these things are true but some of these beliefs are false, especially when it comes to health, and specifically nutrition. Much of the information you read and hear is generalized. Some of the studies you hear about are biased. The party that has the most to gain funds the studies. For instance, the dairy farmers fund many studies that report on the benefits of dairy on bone density. Of course these studies are going to report in favor of dairy. There are a handful of studies out there as well, specifically the Harvard Nurses study, that show no decrease in the incidence of hip and forearm fractures in women who consume milk and other food sources of calcium. (1) Another study suggests that men who drank two or more glasses of milk per day had a greater incidence of prostate cancer. (2) For every study you find in favor of one nutritional theory, you can find another that refutes it. Why is this true? Because we are all unique. I can tell you exactly what I eat that makes me feel the best and you may eat it all and feel absolutely awful. That doesn't make me wrong. That doesn't mean you are making unhealthy decisions. It just means that we each have different things that make us feel good.

For example, maybe one of your beliefs is that you need to eat dairy for calcium and strong bones. Is this really true? Did you know that leafy greens are great sources of calcium? There are 357 mg of calcium in one cup of chopped collard greens and 516 mg of calcium in one bunch of cooked broccoli compared to 290 mg of calcium in one cup of 1% milk. Maybe one of your beliefs is that you have to eat high levels of animal protein in order to become lean. Is that true? What if you are a vegetarian? There are eight grams of protein in a cup of green peas and five grams of protein in a cup of cooked spinach. Or maybe you just finished reading **The China Study** and are starting to question whether a diet high in animal protein is the best choice for you.

In *The China Study*, the research looked at two groups of mice. One group was fed a diet consisting of 10% animal protein and the other group was fed a diet of 30% animal protein (similar to the Standard American Diet). Both groups were then injected with a carcinogen to cause tumors. The 10% group had no sign of tumors in the first, second, or third generation mice. Even in the presence of the carcinogens, they went on to live healthy lives. On the other hand, the 30% animal protein group developed massive tumors, became sickly, and infertile. Of the few second-generation mice that lived, they were full of tumors, very sickly, and infertile. There were no third generation mice. Then, they reversed the diets of the mice. The 10% group, now fed 30% animal protein, grew tumors, became sick and infertile. In the 30% group, now fed 10% animal protein, saw their tumors shrink. They became healthier and regained their fertility. The research identified two groups of humans living in China that follow similar eating patterns of the 10% animal protein group and 30% animal proteins. The study discovered similar occurrences in the humans as occurred in the mice. I share this story not to tell you to stop eating, or even cut back on, your animal protein. I share these findings to point out that many of the beliefs you have about diet and nutrition are simply not true. If you spend your life following every diet you hear about, you will be zigzagging all over. The best thing to do is to experiment with different types of food to determine what works best for you.

Personally, I have never liked meat. If I go to a restaurant, I am much more likely to order fish or a vegetarian dish than I am to order chicken or meat. For many years I forced myself to eat meat because I believed that in order to be lean and strong and to have energy to build the muscle I needed to reach my athletic goals, I had to eat large amounts of meat. Now that I have let go of these beliefs, and choose foods based on what my body needs, I am much healthier and full of energy. I live on a diet of about 10% animal products. This is what I have found works best for me and I found it through experimentation. Occasionally, I do crave meat and I eat it. I feel very good and satisfied when I listen to my body.

(1) Am J Public Health. 1997 Jun;87(6):992-7.**Milk, dietary calcium, and bone fractures in women: a 12-year prospective study.** Feskanich D1, Willett WC, Stampfer MJ, Colditz GA.

(2) Cancer Epidemiol Biomarkers Prev. 2006 Feb;15(2):203-10. **A prospective study of calcium intake and incident and fatal prostate cancer.** Giovannucci E1, Liu Y, Stampfer MJ, Willett WC.

Complete the following exercise to discover which beliefs are holding you back. Refer to the "Limiting Belief Exercise" in the Intuitive Health Workbook.

Write out fifteen beliefs that you have about nutrition, exercise, and health.

Examples:
"No pain. No gain." This is not true. You do not have to hurt to benefit from exercise.

"Healthy food tastes bad." Not true. You just haven't found what you like. Over time your taste buds adjust as your eat whole, unprocessed foods. You body will crave what it needs.

"Exercise is boring." You haven't found that type you enjoy or you're ready for something new.

∾

∾

∾

∾

∾

∾

∾

∾

∾

∾

∾

✧

✧

✧

✧

Write down where you heard each belief. Is it something from your childhood or something you read or heard or something you know from experience?

Put an X through the beliefs that you know are not true.

Circle the beliefs that you question. I encourage you to explore these beliefs.

Re-write a new list of YOUR beliefs about health, food, and exercise.

✧

✧

✧

✧

✧

✧

✧

✧

✧

✧

✧

&

&

&

&

You should now have a deeper understanding of why you eat what you eat and why you are ready to make changes. I hope you realize that your beliefs are not necessarily wrong; they just may not be best for you. In general, a diet comprised primarily of whole foods is healthier than a diet consisting primarily of processed foods. That doesn't mean you have to follow a strict diet and avoid all of the foods that you really enjoy in order to be healthy. I hope you also realize that there is a lot more that goes into great health than just food and exercise. It is not about will power. As you take the first steps to improve your life and health, it will become easier. You will feel the benefits and begin to love yourself.

You now know why it is important to achieve your goals. Now it's time to figure out what changes to make and what areas in your life are out of balance.

Section III

What Should I Change?
What Do I Want to Achieve?

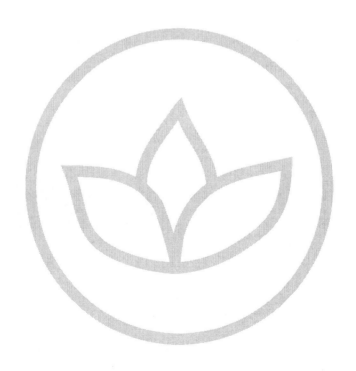

Primary Food

In the previous chapter, you created your definition of health. You learned what it means to you to be healthy. Now that you are aware of what it means to you to be healthy, let's get more specific. Let's figure out what you need to change to get there. When we think of health, we immediately think of exercise and eating healthy food. However, exercise and food are just tools you use to become healthier.

In 1974, Sweden produced the first food pyramid. The United States Department of Agriculture introduced its food pyramid in 1992. This pyramid is the one we most readily think of and recognize. In 2011, the USDA redesigned the pyramid into a plate and named it "My Plate." More easily understood, My Plate is a plate divided into four quarters including vegetables, fruits, grains, and protein, and a serving of dairy on the side. The Integrative Nutrition Plate (IIN Plate) presents an alternative. These diagrams can also be found at www. alligardner.com/bookbonus.

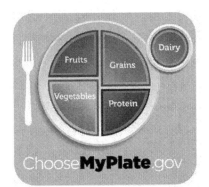 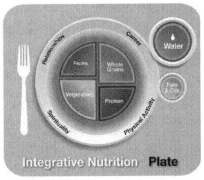

Printed with permission from the Institute of Integrative Nutrition.

There are some similarities between the two diagrams. Both show a plate divided into four quarters, including vegetables, fruit, protein, and whole grains. There are a few differences though. First, the IIN plate is specific about whole grains: leading you to steer away from processed and refined grains that are common in the Standard American Diet. Second, it includes fats and oils, which are extremely important. Thirdly, it has an icon for water. Water is the most important beverage we consume. Dairy is not included in the icon. This is not to say that you should not eat dairy but it is not fundamental in our diet. Lastly, and perhaps most importantly, this icon recognizes that lifestyle plays a crucial role in our health. The outer circle includes: relationships, career, physical activity, and spirituality. This circle symbolizes primary food. Nutrition gives you the fuel to live your life purpose and reach our goals. It is secondary.

Improving your health is not about what foods you eat or how much you weigh or how far you can run or how often you lift weights. Look at the big picture of your life and approach health from the inside out. This journey guides you in discovering what works best for you: your mind, body, and soul.

Circle of Life

A critical aspect of any definition of healthy includes creating balance throughout multiple aspects your life. This is not to say that all aspects have to be evenly balanced and given equal emphasis. When you start putting more emphasis on physical activity and health, you may find that other aspects of your life, such as your career or social life, may receive less emphasis and vice versa. This balance is constantly changing. Just when you think you have balance, it changes. So you must continue to change as well. Let's look at different areas of your life to see where your balance currently lies. This is the circle of life exercise. It is meant to give you a different perspective of your life and areas that may need more attention. Once you have identified the area that needs the most improvement, you will know where your journey begins.

As you look at your life as a whole and focus on the big picture, you will see how every aspect contributes to your health. You can be at your goal weight and be eating all of the "right" things and exercising daily but if you are dissatisfied with your career and financial life you will feel stressed and out of balance. Your dissatisfaction may be interfering with your ability to get a good night's sleep, which may leave you low on energy. Or, you may feel stressed and under a lot of pressure which can cause adrenal fatigue and adversely affect your health. On the other hand, you feel satisfied with your career and financial situation but struggle with your weight. You've directed your time and energy to other aspects of your life. You promise yourself that you'll take care of yourself later. Now, you've dug a hole. It feels too deep to climb out of. You start to improve your health but it is so intimidating you don't know where to begin. You hear stories on the news and gather information on the internet and from magazines. Every expert has a different opinion. You don't know where to start because you don't know what is best for you. You seek out the quick fix and the path of least resistance. This is human nature. However, improving your health will take patience and perseverance. Over time, you will figure out what works best for you and great health will become a great habit. To achieve this though, you have to be willing to work for it and get out of your comfort zone.

Complete the "Circle of Life Exercise" and in the Intuitive Health Workbook to determine which areas of your life are out of balance.

The Circle of Life

Discover which primary foods you are missing, and how to infuse joy and satisfaction into your life.

What does YOUR life look like?

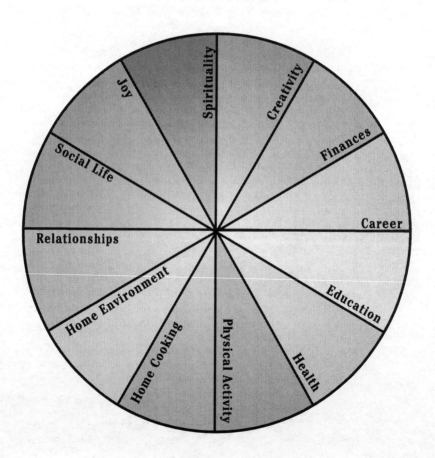

1. Place a dot on the line in each category to indicate your level of satisfaction within each area. Place a dot at the center of the circle to indicate dissatisfaction, or on the periphery to indicate satisfaction. Most people fall somewhere in between.

2. Connect the dots to see your Circle of Life.

3. Identify imbalances. Determine where to spend more time and energy to create balance.

List your top 3 areas that need improvement.

&

&

&

Set SMART Goals

You have to know where you are going; otherwise, how will you ever get there? Often we move through life aimlessly while hoping to be successful. How will you know when you have attained success if you haven't defined it? Many of you have been taught to set goals throughout your life. In elementary school, you set goals to pass your spelling test or sometimes it was to ace your spelling test. In high school, you may have set a goal to make a team, or get a part in the school play, or get into the college you wanted, or to find a job. Maybe you set a goal to find a career that you loved. Maybe you set a goal to find someone to spend your life with and have a family. Maybe you have never really thought about setting goals and if you haven't, this exercise will really stretch you. I encourage you to answer the following questions as truthfully as you can. Remember: this is for you and only you, unless you choose to share it. Since you are reading this book, you most likely have a goal to improve your health.

If you are new to goal setting, let me give you some guidelines that will make your goals more meaningful and productive in reaching them. Set S.M.A.R.T. goals.

Specific. Your goals must be specific and clearly defined.
Measurable. Your goals must be measurable.
Achievable. Your goals must be achievable.
Realistic. Your goals must be realistic.
Timely. Your goals must have a time component.

Examples of SMART goals:
"I will eat at least one serving of greens everyday in January."
"I will engage in physical activity for at least thirty minutes, five days each week."
"I will enjoy a date night with my significant other every other week."
"I will write in my gratitude journal five times each week"

Begin by writing goals to address the area of most dissatisfaction. You may also include overall health goals but make sure they are SMART. Write your six-month goals first. These are your big picture goals. Make sure to take into account your WHY. Next, write your three-month goals keeping your six-month goals in mind. What do you need to do to be on track to achieve your six-month goals? Finally, write your one-month goals. These are changes and steps you can start today to get you moving in the right direction.

Use the "SMART Goals Worksheet" in the Intuitive Health Workbook to define your goals. Write these goals down on a piece of paper and place them so that you will see them every day to motivate and remind you what you are working towards.

As you write you goals, make sure to address Primary and Secondary Foods.

6 Month Goals

∽

∽

∽

Three Month Goals

∽

∽

∽

One Month Goals

∽

∽

∽

Create Your Vision

You have identified your goals for the next 90 days. You have a deeper understanding of how to achieve them. Your work thus far has uncovered many of the underlying thoughts and behaviors that have prevented you from achieving your goals. Next, create your vision for your health. Use the "Creating Your Life purpose" and "Vision Exercise" found in the Intuitive Health Workbook.

If you don't know where you are going, how will you ever get there?

The first step to create your vision is to determine what you value most in life. What is most important to you? If you create a vision that is not in line with your values, then you will either never attain your vision or you will be incredibly unhappy getting there. Right now, create a list of the top five things you value most in life. Some possibilities for your list: time for family, loyalty, honesty, health, integrity, freedom, activity, creating things, teamwork, independence, generosity, security.

What do you value most?

❧

❧

❧

❧

❧

The second step is to determine your life purpose. As I discussed in the introduction, health is not just about what we eat, how much we exercise, or how much we weigh. Health is integral to being truly happy. Health is about having the energy, strength, wisdom, and mindset to be the best you. Health is about finding balance and creating harmony in every aspect of your life.

Let's define your life purpose.
What are you great at?

What things do you look forward to doing every day?

Name three things that come naturally and easily to you.

If you could do anything, be anything, what would it be?

This exercise may stretch you a little and that's okay. You may not feel totally clear on your life purpose. Your life purpose may evolve and change as you grow and develop a greater awareness and understanding. Your life purpose is much greater than your job or career.

Create a life purpose statement that sums up who you are and what you are meant to be.

Create your life vision. Include every aspect of your life, from your health and wellness, to your relationships, your career, and your spirituality. Be as detailed as you can be. Use all of your senses as you create your vision. What do you look like? Where are you? What does it feel like to be you? What feelings do you give off to others who are around you? What do you sound like? How do you talk to yourself? How do you talk to others? What do others say about you? What do you smell when you vision your life? What does it taste like to be you?

Using these details, **write out a detailed ten-year vision**. Where do you see yourself in ten years? What is your ideal life? Anything is possible. You have all of the resources, time, money, and support. What do you truly desire?

Next, keeping your ten-year vision in mind, **write out your three-year vision**. What things must happen in three years for you to be on track to reach your ten-year vision?

Finally, **make a list of goals you would like to achieve in the next year** to be on track to achieve your three year and ten year visions.

Create your vision in detail. What will you look like, what will your life look like, and what will it feel like to reach your health goals?

Looking far ahead is difficult. What if you don't achieve your vision? You may have a fear of setting yourself up for failure. Or, maybe you really haven't thought about it and you don't know what your vision is.

I'm not a fortuneteller but I have a very clear vision of where I am headed. I don't know exactly where I'll be in ten years but I know where I would like to be. My vision is clear and in line with my values and my life purpose. The purpose of this exercise is not to predict the future but to set you in a path of becoming a better, more fulfilled version of you. Health issues arise from living a life that is not in alignment with our values and life purpose. Your body works to achieve homeostasis, the physiological term for balance. If you are out of balance or not living a life in line with your values, you create stress. If you do not handle stress appropriately, health issues suddenly loom large. Once you get clear on your values, life purpose, and vision, you will begin to experience true health and happiness.

Make your vision visible in whatever medium works best for you. Write out statements on note cards and set them in places you will frequently read them. Create a vision board that you place where you see it throughout the day. Generate a vision statement to say to yourself every night before you go to sleep. There is no right answer. The key is that you see, hear, and feel your vision daily. You re-program your subconscious to believe your vision to be true. This is the next step. Own your vision until it is reality.

You defined goals that you would like to achieve in the course of the next year to bring you one step closer to your vision. Now it's time to take action to make those goals a reality.

Section IV

How Do I actually Make Changes in My Habits and Health?

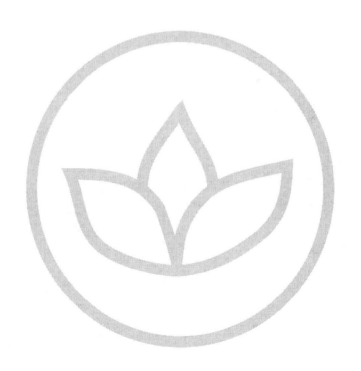

Take Action

You have determined why you want to improve your health and what areas you want to improve. It is now time to make a plan, put your plan into action, and follow through. This is where we get stuck. This is what we think of as the difficult part. Let's keep it simple and manageable. Transforming your health and your habits requires time. Change doesn't happen overnight. We set unrealistic expectations and are disappointed when we don't achieve our goals. We give up because we aren't making progress fast enough so we look for a better, faster path. Remember: the goal is to make great health a great habit. It is a process of trial and error. It is not about being perfect. You will learn much more from your mistakes than your accomplishments. Give yourself permission to make mistakes, but learn from them. When astronauts set off for the moon, they know their destination. Along the way, they make thousands of course changes. These changes are necessary to keep them on course to their final destination. There is not a direct course or a right way to achieve your vision.

Here are some steps to put your plan in action.

- ✑ **Make a plan.**
- ✑ **Add it in.**
- ✑ **Be accountable.**
- ✑ **Correlate your behaviors and outcomes.**

1. Make a plan

No matter what your goal is or what behavior you are changing, you have to start with a plan. Make adjustments as you go but start with a plan. Your plan doesn't have to be perfect and it will change as you move forward.

One question asked daily is, "What am I going to eat?" We all face it, usually three to five times every day. Without planning, you find yourself staring into the pantry or refrigerator trying to decide what to eat. Unhealthy decisions occur in these moments especially if you haven't been grocery shopping recently. There is nothing to eat. It is six o'clock. You are hungry. Your kids are hungry and your best and easiest choice is to go out. Sometimes you can make a good decision and find a healthy option. However, food prepared at home is almost always healthier, not to mention less expensive. Make a plan. Figure out what works best for you and your life.

If you enjoy planning, you may like to sit down once a week before you head out the door to the grocery store. If you don't like planning, you can create a monthly plan and then make small adjustments as things come up. Start with looking at your calendar for the week. Write down all of the activities and events for the week. Then fill in meals accordingly. If you are working late on Thursday or your kids have a soccer game Tuesday night, you will want to plan for a meal that is quick to prepare or maybe something in the crockpot so the prep is in the morning and your meal is ready for you when you get home. I keep a list of meals my family enjoys next to me as I fill in the calendar. It makes for a great reference and I don't have to reinvent the wheel each time I meal plan. Once you decide on the meals for the week make a grocery list. There are many apps out there that can help make this process easier too. Once you have a system in place, meal planning will become a habit and you will be more prepared to make great food choices. Schedule time to go to the grocery store and to prepare your meals.

The same idea holds true with exercise. You have to schedule it and make it a priority otherwise it does not happen. Decide what you like to do and make a plan to do it. Personally, I do best when I exercise in the morning. When I am consistent, it's easier to get going because it becomes a habit. Also, scheduling times to meet a friend, go to an exercise class, or meet a trainer or coach makes it easier to be consistent. But, you must have a plan and set aside time to carry it out.

2. Add it in

When starting a diet, we immediately think about all of the yummy food we won't be able to eat. We think: no more carbs, no more sugar, no more caffeine, no more of the good stuff. Right away, those thoughts fill us with dread and negative feelings toward our new diet. We know it's going to be all about will power. We may stay the course for a while but eventually we fall off the wagon and revert to our old ways. Then we are angry and disappointed that we weren't strong enough to stay the course. We failed. We gave into a lack of willpower. Diets are viewed as a short-term solution and abandoned once a goal is met or the going gets tough.

Instead, focus on adding in new foods and behaviors. When you add in more healthy foods and habits, you will crowd out your old unhealthy habits. You create lifelong sustainable habits that become integral in your life. Learn to enjoy delicious food that provides nutrition and satisfies your needs. Focus on positive habits and those that make you happy and healthy. As you make health a priority, your outlook changes. Rather than beating yourself up for eating chocolate cake, celebrate all of the healthy things you ate. Celebrate every vegetable, piece of fruit, and glass of water that you consumed today. Make note of how great your body feels for each of these things. It is not a game of willpower. Add in exercise because it makes you feel good and energized. Set yourself up to succeed right from the start. Put your energy and attention towards the behaviors that make you feel your best. Build yourself up and celebrate each step. Acknowledge each time you make a great health decision and be proud that you are moving one step closer to your goal.

You may currently drink soda every day. Instead of drinking soda, add in more glasses of water. You will quench your thirst and thus reduce the amount of soda you drink, without relying on your will power. The more greens you eat, the more you will enjoy them and want them. Five years ago, if someone asked me to drink the green smoothie I drink today, I probably would have hated it. Now, I crave them. Give yourself time. Changes in health and the foods you eat do not change overnight. When you reshape your nutrition overnight, it becomes overwhelming. Add in one healthy behavior at a time. Revisit the Circle of Life exercise in Chapter 8 and focus on the area of Primary Food that may be affecting your health.

As a culture, we are obsessed with counting calories. We have been taught that in order to lose weight, you need to consume fewer calories than you expend. However, the quality of the food you consume is much more important. A calorie is a measure of energy. The way our body processes food is very different based on the type of calories you consume. When you eat foods that are high in vitamins and minerals and fiber and low in sugar, your body uses all of those nutrients and remains satiated for a longer period of time. When you eat foods high in sugar and refined carbohydrates, your body requires more food to meet your nutritional requirements. You also have a spike in blood sugar. There are addictive behaviors that are linked to diets high in sugar. You can eat a meal high in calories from a fast food restaurant and still be hungry an hour later. On the other hand, you can eat a meal that has fewer calories and remain full for hours.

This is not a lesson in calorie counting. When you choose to eat higher quality food, you will feel better. Instead of creating a list of foods you can eat and foods you cannot, consider creating a set of guidelines to follow. These are not fast rules, but guidelines to your nutrition. Strive to make great food choices 90% of the time. This sounds like a high number to strive for but it is very manageable.

A typical day includes three meals and two snacks. If you eat breakfast at home every morning and make healthy snacks readily accessible, you will have managed 60% of your meals. It is easier to make healthy decisions at home than at a restaurant. Weekday lunches can be primarily leftovers or a green smoothie. Dinner is the last meal to worry about and the one most frequently eaten at a restaurant. If you make great nutritional decisions in four of seven dinners, you can be flexible with the other three. Let go of the guilt around food. It is just food. It is not worth beating yourself up over. When you make a poor decision and eat too much or eat something unhealthy, recognize that you made a poor decision and move on. Commit to making a better decision at the very next meal.

Create a new habit of great health. Add in positive behaviors to improve your health. The more you implement these positive behaviors into daily life, the more you crowd out behaviors that make you feel unhealthy. A habit is an action that we perform automatically without thinking about it. Habits are triggered by cues and lead to rewards. For instance, you might have a habit of drinking coffee in the morning. The cue is that you wake up, use the bathroom, and head for the coffee pot. The reward is the burst of energy from the caffeine, the feeling of warmth, and the enjoyment of the morning ritual. Often the reward has a physical, mental, and emotional component. Habits are formed through repetition. Once you have formed a habit, it requires less energy, less attention, and less brain activity to perform. Here are some examples.

Every morning, you have rituals that you perform. You wake up, get out of bed, go to the bathroom, have a cup of coffee, and read the newspaper. You go through the motions without even thinking about what you are doing. I have been drinking a smoothie for breakfast for almost seven years. I don't even think about it anymore. I put all of the ingredients into my blender and blend. I'm on autopilot. It's quick and easy and works for me.

Create new habits for your daily routine with the "Daily Habits Worksheet" found in the Intuitive Health Workbook.

Make a list of those things that you do almost every day, i.e. your morning routine.

Next, identify which habits are improving your health and those that are detrimental.
List three new healthy habits to implement this week.

୶

୶

୶

We also have habits around eating our meals. When you sit down to eat a meal, you can only eat so much before you feel full. Your stomach has a maximum capacity. Often, you don't listen to the stomach's message because you are distracted and eating for the sake of eating. Instead, start with your favorite foods and the healthiest choices. Fill up on veggies, lean protein, and whole foods rather than bread. When you start to feel full put your fork down.

My kids usually start whining and snacking as I'm making dinner. Instead of letting them fill up on crackers and snacks, I put a plate of veggies or edamame on the table. Even though they are snacking, I know they're filling up on the good stuff. Make it a habit to eat the healthy foods first and stop eating when you are full.

The same is true with liquid. The general recommendation is to drink half of your body weight (in pounds) in ounces of water each day. If you aren't used to drinking water, half of your body weight in ounces is a lot of water. In addition, if you are drinking three or more sodas a day, you may struggle to drink that much liquid. The next time you find yourself reaching for a soda, drink a glass of water first. Then, if you still want the soda, go ahead and drink it but you will probably drink less because you will be full of water. Keep up this habit of water first and over time you will find that you will drink more water and less soda. This works great with sweets, too. Next time you crave something sweet, like chocolate, drink a glass of water instead. If you still want that chocolate, take a bite and enjoy it. The first two bites are always the best and then stop. Over time you will create a habit of eating less of the foods that you are trying to avoid.

As you become more mindful of your behaviors, you will identify keystone habits. A keystone habit is something you do that triggers a series of other behaviors. All behaviors connect to each other. This can be either a positive or a negative. For instance, a keystone habit may be exercising first thing in the morning. Early morning exercise may leave you energized and feeling organized and productive. You feel like you begin the day having already accomplished a lot. It may motivate you to eat a healthy breakfast, which then gives you the energy and focus to be productive at work. You may then eat a healthy lunch, wanting to stay on track and keep feeling good. This may continue throughout the rest of your day. You go to sleep early so you get adequate rest in order to wake early again to exercise. See how the keystone habit of exercising triggers a cascade of other healthy choices and behaviors. Another example of a keystone habit may be eating a great breakfast. Starting your day off with a solid meal leaves you energized and focused at work. It is easier to make healthy decisions and maintain portion control when you are not famished. It is important for you to identify your keystone habit. Once you identify it, make sure to integrate this habit into your daily routine and other healthy routines will follow. On the other hand, a keystone habit may be waking up late in the morning and rushing through your morning routine. This causes you to skip breakfast. At lunch you eat more than you would like which leaves you low on energy in the afternoon. You leave work with the intention of going to exercise but you find that you are too tired and vow to exercise tomorrow. Then you feel down on yourself for not exercising another day and eat to make you feel better. A poor food choice at dinner may disrupt your sleep leaving you too tired to wake up early the next morning. You now see how our behaviors feed off of each other.

Identify one positive keystone habit to implement into your morning routine. It may be exercise, it might be to eat a healthy breakfast, it might be to spend 10 minutes writing in your journal and setting an intention for your day. Pick something that will improve your day.

3. Be accountable.

You have a plan. You are creating new habits. Now follow through with your plan. You may be highly motivated and disciplined at times while struggling at other moments. You have to set up a system to hold yourself accountable. First, determine whether you will be accountable to yourself or someone else. Having a support system in place will help. Find a coach, a friend, a co-worker, or a family member to help you succeed. Second, schedule specific times to check in and review your accomplishments and goals. This way you will be able to celebrate your accomplishments and see what you need to improve on. This also allows you to set new goals or to adjust your plan to continue moving forward. Finally, make your goals and action steps visible. Clearly post your steps in a place where you will see them every day, it may be on your refrigerator, your bathroom mirror, or your calendar. This will serve as a reminder to keep you on track. Determine the best way to hold yourself accountable. Do you thrive on lists? Do you prefer to have a support system to check in with? Do you enjoy the feeling of success when you follow through?

4. Correlate your behaviors and outcomes.

You won't always follow your plan exactly. You will eat too much. You will skip your daily exercise. You will eat food that you know doesn't make you feel good. Although you don't have to beat yourself up, you do need to recognize how your decisions and actions make you feel. Until you correlate your feelings with your actions, you will continue to make the same decisions; thus, have the same outcome. The food you eat affects you physically, mentally, and emotionally.

For years I experienced bloating and stomach pain everyday around lunchtime. I ate a healthy breakfast of oatmeal with skim milk and fruit almost every morning. Then, on my way to work, I stopped for a vanilla latte. I believed that I needed calcium and protein from dairy products. I continued this behavior for years not correlating the two behaviors: too much cow's milk caused bloating and stomach pain. When I did make the connection, I sought alternatives for breakfast. I begin drinking a cup of coffee instead of a latte. I used almond milk in my oatmeal instead of cow's milk. I began to feel much better throughout the day.

I worked with a client who struggled with low energy in the middle of the day. She was training for a triathlon. She scheduled her workouts for the early morning. She rarely made time for breakfast prior to her workouts but ate some fruit after her workouts. She had a salad for lunch in the early afternoon. The majority of her meals were eaten out. She rarely bought food at the grocery store to have on hand. She did not correlate that her low calorie intake in the morning combined with intense exercise contributed to her low energy in the afternoon. Once we increased her calories in the morning around her exercise, her mid-afternoon energy improved.

As you begin to add different foods to your diet, listen to how your body feels with each food. It is important to correlate the foods you eat with how you feel. Identify times when you eat for the sake of eating rather than to fuel and nourish your body. Your moods can trigger eating habits. Do you reach for food at certain times of the day even though you are not hungry? You also may be eating foods that may or may not work for your body. You may have difficulty digesting certain foods. When you have sensitivity to a food, your body may have excessive inflammation as a result. This may lead to digestive problems, respiratory problems, and other illness due to a weakened immune system. It is important to spend time to figure out what foods work best for your body. Explore a variety of exercises to help you correlate your behaviors and outcomes on pages 51 and 52.

Your body communicates with you in the form of cravings. We are programmed to believe that cravings are bad. We learn this because the things we crave most are sugar and salt, which are both things we are taught to avoid. We hear that we have too much sodium and sugar in our diets, primarily a product of too much processed food. However, when you stop to listen, you will find that you crave things that are great for you, too. Your body is an amazing instrument. Your body knows how to maintain homeostasis. Your body knows when to go to sleep and when to wake up and when it is time to use the bathroom. It is your job to listen to these signals. Automatically, your body maintains a body temperature of 98.6 degrees and repairs itself when it is wounded. Your heart continually beats. Your lungs automatically inhale oxygen. Your body is an amazing computer that rarely makes a mistake. You need to listen to your body, not what your brain is telling you.

Your body sends messages to you to assist you in maintaining balance. These messages come in the form of cravings. It is your job to deconstruct those cravings and figure out what your body needs. Cravings are not a sign of weakness. Cravings are a signal that your body needs something. There are six primary causes of cravings.

   Lack of primary food. When you are unhappy with your current life situation, you crave food and use food to make you feel better. This is emotional eating. You eat out of boredom or when you are stressed. If you are dissatisfied in a relationship or uninspired with your current job you may look to food for entertainment or to fill the void. When you lack an appropriate exercise routine or a spiritual practice, you may turn to food to fill the void of primary food. Look at different areas of your life to see where you can improve. As you improve these areas, how you view food changes too.

   Water. Thirst is frequently misinterpreted for hunger. When you lack adequate water intake, you feel thirsty before becoming dehydrated. Dehydration is manifested as mild hunger. Instead of snacking, drink a full glass of water next time a craving strikes. If you are still hungry, then eat a healthy snack.

   Your past. You are shaped by your childhood and past experiences. Your body remembers foods you ate and the emotions and feelings associated with them. You crave foods to reproduce those feelings.

   Seasonal. Food cravings can be brought on by the season. In the winter, we crave hot, comfort foods. As mammals, we naturally hibernate and store fat in the winter. In the spring, we emerge and become more active. Eating leafy greens helps us to detoxify from our winter habits. Eating seasonal fruits and vegetables maintains your connection with the earth.

෴ **Lack of nutrients.** When you are low in nutrients, your body craves food to replenish the nutrients. A craving for ice cream may be a sign that you need more fat in your diet. A craving for seaweed may be a sign that you are low in iodine.

෴ **Hormonal.** Our hormone levels are constantly in flux. Cravings that occur monthly or cyclically may be related to hormones. Make healthy choices to satisfy your cravings.

When you try to avoid something, it becomes your primary focus. The more you think about it, the more it consumes your thoughts, and the more difficult it becomes to avoid. Instead of avoiding your cravings, figure out why you have the craving. Here are four tips to help you manage your cravings.

෴ Have a glass of water and wait ten minutes. If the craving persists, then have some of whatever you are craving.

෴ Eat a healthier version of what you crave. For example, if you crave sweets, try eating more fruit and sweet or root vegetables.

෴ Examine what is going on in your life. Identify the cause of your craving.

෴ When you eat the food you are craving, enjoy it, taste it, savor it. Notice its effect. Next time, you will become more aware and free to decide if you really want it.

How Do You Make Changes?

You now have an understanding of why you want to be healthy and what it will mean to you and your loved ones. You know which areas of your life are not in balance and need some extra attention. You have created a vision and know what you would like your life to look like and feel like. You have learned the importance of making a plan and sticking to it. Now is the time to take action and figure out how to make these changes. How are you going to change your life? How will you implement long-term, healthy habits that will shape the rest of your life?

Health books are a billion dollar industry. Each one claims that it holds the key to improving your life and trimming your waistline. Occasionally, you might find one that fits and works for you. You may follow its rules and guidelines for a while but when your body and life shift, the guidelines no longer fit. You go in search of the next book that will give you the new answers. Wouldn't it be nice if you developed an understanding of your own body and what you need to do to maintain your health? That is my intention. I want us to create a blueprint together for you to follow for the rest of your life. This blueprint will be specific to you, yet flexible, and allows you to enjoy your life and all that it offers. There are no hard rules, just guidelines that you strive to live by. Over time, they become easier, and they occur without much thought. As you learn to listen to your body, you will discover that you hold the answers to your health.

How you become healthy is unique to you, and only you know the path. The foods I eat and the foods I feed my children seem to be highly scrutinized by those around me since I am a health coach. At a party, a woman looked at my plate and asked me if I was really going to eat the pita bread with the hummus. I replied, "I'll try it. If it tastes good today, I'll eat it, if not I'll leave it on my plate." I have tried the highly restrictive diets. I frequently found myself in situations where none of the food available was on my list of acceptable foods so I would choose to not eat. However, as a mother of three, I have been pregnant or breastfeeding the majority of the last eight years. Skipping meals was detrimental. Without enough nutrition, my energy levels plummeted and I found myself frequently sick. When I ate, I was eating the right things but it led to a feast or famine situation. Now, I strive to make the best decision with what is presented to me. If we eat out at a restaurant, I make the best food choice I can. I always eat my favorite foods first and leave food on my plate when I feel satisfied. This is portion control. This doesn't mean that I only eat a fist-sized portion of meat. It means that some nights, my body may need a little more meat so I listen. I may have less rice to compensate. But I give my body what it is asking for. My vegetables are the first things to be eaten. They have become my favorite.

The rest of this chapter focuses on different tools you can use to help you connect with your mind, body, and soul. These exercises will challenge you to improve your intuition. Once you complete one or all of these experiments, you will better understand what foods make you feel great and which foods you should limit or avoid. Your body and your nutritional needs are constantly changing. It is important to listen and continually adapt your diet.

Journaling

A great tool to correlate behaviors is journaling. I like to begin each journal entry with a list of five things I am grateful for. This shifts my focus to the positive and I find my entries are more productive. Write whatever comes to mind. Have a dialogue with yourself. Write things that are going on both good and bad. Write your successes, failures, struggles, and solutions. Write down your actions and outcomes. Then, write down how you will do it differently next time. Over time, you will recognize patterns and behaviors that you repeat and their eventual outcomes. Create a habit of journaling every morning or at least a few times each week. Keep your writing positive. Recognize the changes you want to make. Acknowledge the poor decisions. Focus on the outcomes and the changes you will make to do it better next time.

Food mood journal

This a combination of your journal and a food log. In a notebook, write down everything you eat and the time. Next to each entry write down how you feel physically and emotionally before, during, and after each thing you eat. Keeping a food diary is a great tool to make the connections between the foods you eat and how you feel. It is a great place to learn if you eat out of boredom or because you are trying to fill a void in your life with food. Listen to your body. This is an opportunity for you to learn from your body and help you improve the decisions you make.

Breakfast experiment

Each morning for one week, eat a different meal but keep it simple. Write down what you ate and how you felt right after eating and two hours later. Pay attention to your energy levels, your mood, your physical symptoms, and your level of satisfaction. Examples of daily food choices are: eggs, bacon or sausage or tofu, oatmeal or any grain product, boxed breakfast cereal, muffin and coffee, fresh fruit, and fresh vegetables. Experimenting with breakfast foods gives you a clean slate to learn how your body reacts to certain foods, since you have fasted all night. After experimenting with different foods, you will have a better understanding of what you enjoy eating and what makes you feel best.

Elimination diet

For two weeks, eliminate all foods that you suspect make you feel bad. These foods most commonly include but are not limited to gluten, dairy, soy, nuts, and eggs. You can eliminate them all at once or one at a time. After two weeks, add each food back into your diet one at a time, three days apart. Notice how you feel, once you add the food back into your diet. For this to work, you must completely eliminate the food. Read labels closely for hidden sources. You may be surprised to learn what is actually in the foods you eat. For the two weeks, your diet will consist of primarily whole foods. Once you know which foods are making you sick, you may then choose to eliminate them entirely or eat them in moderation based on what your body tolerates.

Create a nutrition blueprint

A nutrition blueprint is a set of guidelines that you follow as you make food choices. It is not meant to be a set of hard and fast rules that you follow to a T. Use the "Nutrition Blueprint Guide" in the Intuitive Health Workbook.

Here is my nutrition blueprint. These are the general guidelines that I follow.

    ∽   Strive for healthy, nutrient dense meals 90% of the time;

- ✑ Focus on whole foods – fruits, veggies, nuts, seeds, legumes, fats, lean animal protein;
- ✑ Eat my favorite foods first at every meal and stop eating when I'm full;
- ✑ Choose organic when possible, especially with the dirty dozen plus (includes apples, strawberries,
- ✑ Gapes, celery, peaches, spinach, sweet bell peppers, nectarines, cucumbers, cherry tomatoes, snap peas, and potatoes. Also, hot peppers and blueberries);
- ✑ Select grass fed, hormone free animal products;
- ✑ Eat nitrate free meats;
- ✑ Avoid cow's milk in favor of alternatives– coconut, almond, rice, etc.;
- ✑ Avoid Trans Fats and high fructose corn syrup;
- ✑ Eat only when I'm hungry, when in doubt, I drink a glass of water;
- ✑ Prepare the majority of meals at home;
- ✑ Drink a green smoothie or fresh juice everyday;
- ✑ Listen to my body before I eat to determine what I really want;
- ✑ Minimize added sugar intake;
- ✑ Look for whole food ingredients and avoid enriched ingredients;
- ✑ No soda pop;
- ✑ Remember: food is just food.

I don't count calories. I don't worry about percentages of proteins and carbs, and fats. I listen to my body and feed it what it needs. I eat my favorite foods first, then when I'm full and I look down at my plate I see foods that I don't really love. This makes it easier to leave food on my plate when I have had enough. When I am craving something, I look for the reason behind my cravings. When I was pregnant with my third child, I craved red meat. I had never enjoyed red meat prior to this period. I ate red meat because my body needed more iron or protein from the meat than I was getting from my normal diet. I avoid highly processed foods. I focus on whole foods, including fresh vegetables and fruits. I drink water. I also drink coffee and wine. I make the best decision with the choices I have in front of me.

These guidelines have become habits. Over time, you will create your own guidelines. You will create a blueprint to live by. It is important that your guidelines are not too stringent otherwise you will face constant failure. When I began my journey to learn about and embrace nutrition, my list was very different. I made one change at a time. When I tried to jump too far ahead, I became discouraged and overwhelmed. I currently feel stronger and healthier than any other point in my life. I exercise less but have a greater sense of balance and harmony in my life.

Section V

Knowledge is Power

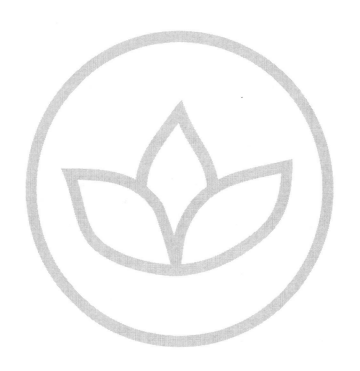

Section Five is divided up into chapters focusing on how to improve your health and happiness. There is no direct or correct path. I encourage you to start with the chapters that will give you the greatest success and create a foundation, such as incorporating greens and water into your daily diet. Next, address the area that is most out of balance and needs attention in your life. This may be exercise, self care, career, and/or relationships. Read the chapter, work through the questions, and then implement the steps into your life, one at a time. Each step builds on the prior one. Continue to implement each step until you have addressed them all. You determine the timeline. Some steps may be easier than others and some may already be a habit in your life.

This section is divided into the following topics:
    Greens
    Water
    Exercise
    Grains
    Self Care
    Protein
    Posture
    Fats
    Sleep
    Portion Control
    Healthy Snacking
    Controversial Foods
    Detoxify Your Home

Glorious Greens

Greens play a vital role in our health. The Standard American Diet (SAD) is missing this vital component to health. The average diet is severely lacking green vegetables. When you create a habit of adding daily greens to your diet you naturally begin to crowd out many of the foods that make you sick. Let's start with the benefits of greens and then we'll move into some suggestions of how you can add them into your daily nutrition.

What are greens? The most common is probably broccoli but others include but are not limited to spinach, kale, bok choy, collards, watercress, mustard greens, cabbage, arugula, endive, Swiss chard, and many others. Greens are very high in vitamins and minerals including calcium, magnesium, iron, potassium, phosphorus, zinc, and vitamins A, C, E, and K. They are also loaded with fiber, folic acid, chlorophyll, and many other micronutrients. Some of the health benefits associated with consuming dark, leafy, green vegetables are cancer prevention, improved circulation, strengthened immune system, promotion of healthy intestinal flora, improved energy, improved function of vital organs, and cleared congestion. (IIN)

How do you incorporate greens into your daily diet? In my opinion, the easiest and fastest way is through the green smoothie. By creating a smoothie of greens and fruits, you get a meal that is jam packed with nutrients. It's also an easier and incredibly convenient way to get your greens. You need ten minutes to put it all in a blender and mix it up. You can take a smoothie anywhere.

What do you need? First you need a commercial grade blender. If your blender isn't powerful enough to breakdown all of the ingredients, the smoothie won't be very appetizing. Second, you need water, greens, and fruit. Here's my favorite recipe:

2 C water
3-4 big handfuls of greens
1 banana
1-2 C frozen fruit
1 apple
¼ lemon (with skin for antioxidants)

The more fruit you add the sweeter it will be. As you first start with the green smoothie habit, use more fruit. As your taste buds change as you add more green to your diet, then you can add less fruit. Aim for 50-50 ratios, or even more greens depending on your personal preference. If you don't like the green smoothie, try again with a different combination of fruit. Blending, unlike juicing, retains the fiber from the fruit, which helps balance your blood sugar. If you need more fruit to make it palatable, add it.

You can also add in a daily green salad. Focus on dark, leafy greens. You can be creative and add any topping you choose. Cut-up veggies, fruit, nuts, seeds, dried fruit, lean protein are all great choices. As for salad dressing, homemade is always best. Olive oil and balsamic vinegar is an easy option. If you are hooked on other commercially prepared salad dressings that's okay. Just try to use a little less. As your taste buds get more accustomed to the taste of greens, you will want less and less dressing.

Action step:

    ✍ **Add in a green smoothie or green salad every day.**

Water

Your body is composed primarily of water. You need water to function. You can only survive without water for three days. Most people don't drink enough water. How much water to drink is one of the most frequently asked questions. The answer is that it depends. If you are thirsty then you are already in a state of dehydration. A general rule of thumb for water intake is to drink half of your body weight (in pounds) in ounces of water each day. So, if I weigh 130 pounds then my goal should be 65 ounces of water each day. There are a lot of variables that can affect this but this a great starting point. For instance, your water needs will increase as your activity level increases, in hotter weather, in dryer climates. Your water levels will also fluctuate based on hormones, illness, and stress. You need to listen to your body. The next time you are craving sweets, try drinking a glass of water instead. Keep in mind that cravings for sugar are misinterpreted for dehydration.

Action step:

ﻼ **Drink half of your body weight (in pounds) in ounces of water each day this week.**

Exercise

What are you feeling as I begin the topic of exercise? Are you excited to see what new ideas I offer to motivate you to continue? Do you sense anxiety or guilt because exercise is something you know you are supposed to do but you don't? Are you apprehensive because you've tried to exercise but you never stick with it and you feel like a failure?

What is exercise? What is it about exercise that makes it so difficult to be consistent? Most likely, it's because you don't like what you're doing. You have created an idea of what you have to do based on things you have been told, things you have heard, or things you have read. But, like nutrition, exercise is not a one-size-fits-all thing. What you like to do, what works best for your body, and the amount of time you are willing to spend are all very individual matters. It is also dynamic and your exercise needs change over time. If you're not used to exercising or if you do not feel comfortable in your own skin, beginning an exercise program is a challenge. You don't know what to do. You feel uncomfortable. You don't want to get hurt. You dread exercising. You procrastinate and use every excuse in the book to get out of it. Then you feel guilty that another day has passed without starting your exercise program.

How many times have you made a New Year's resolution to exercise more? The most common New Year's Resolution is to lose weight. Losing weight frequently involves diet and exercise. My intention is to shed light on a different way to approach exercise. It doesn't have to be something you dread and it definitely shouldn't make you feel bad. Let's break it down and make exercise more enjoyable.

Don't do it because you have to, do it because you love it! -
Anonymous

Why should you exercise? There are many medically proven results of exercise. Consistent exercise helps to control weight, lowers blood pressure, enhances quality sleep, improves mood, decreases the incidence of heart disease, improves balance and coordination, improves immune function, improves flexibility, decreases fatty liver disease, improves bone density, increases energy, and improves cognitive function. What about all of the other reasons to exercise? Exercise also improves your mood, your self-esteem, your posture, and your general feeling of well being. What if you changed your thought process around exercise? What if you began to exercise because you loved it? Because it made you feel good? What if exercise became something you looked forward to everyday because you enjoyed it, and loved how it made you feel instead of exercising because someone told you that you have to exercise in order to lose weight? What if you could do any kind of physical activity you enjoyed, and what if your exercise could change daily or weekly based or your mood and energy? Would you look forward to exercise as something you got to do rather than dreading it and putting it off as long as you could or avoiding it entirely? Has it ever crossed your mind that maybe you just haven't found the right exercise for you??

What is exercise exactly, and what activities count as exercise? Let's start with the definition. Exercise is physical activity that is performed with the goal of improving or sustaining your health.

That's pretty broad. It doesn't say that you have to be drenched in sweat or run for miles to exercise. It doesn't say anywhere that you have to exercise for at least thirty minutes for it to count. Nor does it say that you have to do cross fit or boot camp or a spinning class for it to count as daily exercise. We impose these beliefs about exercise on ourselves. We watch the Biggest Loser and think that we have to exercise to the point of absolute exhaustion. We force ourselves to run because we can burn the most calories that way or we see a runner who is fit and healthy and think that's what we have to do.

We are all unique. We all have different goals. Our goals change as we go through life. Therefore, we should all exercise in a mode that is unique to us and makes us feel good. Exercise habits and routines will change throughout your life. Just because you used to love to run or push yourself to the extremes doesn't mean that's what you should be doing now. Listen to your body. Find what's best for you.

How do you know what to do? Follow the same four guidelines presented in Chapter 10 starting on page 36. Those guidelines are:

✎ **Make a plan / What do you like to do?**

✎ **Add it in / Schedule it;**

✎ **Be accountable;**

✎ **Correlate your behaviors and outcomes.**

I encourage you to re-read that section.

1. Pick an activity that you are excited about and you want to do

What do you love to do you? What makes you excited to get moving? Is it a hike in the mountains, an exercise class with a friend, a Pilates class, a walk with your dog, yoga, or a solitary run to be lost in your thoughts? It doesn't really matter what you choose to do, just that you choose to do something to move your body. Try something new. Answer the following questions to determine what type of exercise you enjoy the most.

Whom? What? Where? When? Why?

Whom do you like to exercise with? Are you motivated by the presence of others? Do you love the feeling of being pushed by a coach or an instructor or trainer? Do you prefer to exercise alone? There is no one correct answer. It might even change from day to day. Some days you might thrive on the comraderie of working out with others and love to know that you are all in the same place working towards similar goals. You may find it inspiring. It might help you get there because you know you are meeting someone. Other days, you might love the idea of spending time alone with your thoughts. You might enjoy listening to your body and just moving and doing what feels best that day.

What do you enjoy doing? I have worked with many people struggling with their weight who tell me that they hate to exercise. I believe they just haven't found what they love to do. They have limited themselves into believing that they have to move a certain way or do a specific type of exercise to see results. They drag themselves to the gym, hating every minute, and spend a long time on the elliptical because they think that's what they have to do. I would probably hate exercise, too.

Sometimes you get excited and motivated about exercise. You go to the gym and start lifting weights and doing cardio. You work with a personal trainer or go to some classes. You go all in and beat yourself up thinking that's what exercise is all about. "No pain, no gain" right? Then you feel so miserable you don't ever want to go back. You give up before you ever get to the good part when you walk out of the gym feeling energized like you've just done something great for your body. Many people never get to that point.

We are not all built the same. Our bodies respond differently to different types of exercise. If you are new to exercise, experiment with different types until you find what you love. If you have been exercising awhile but are now plateauing and not seeing the results you once did, mix it up and attempt something new. Whenever you begin a new exercise program or routine, the greatest results are seen in the first four weeks. This is when neurological adaptation occurs. You become stronger and faster and feel your endurance improve. You are not actually gaining more muscle. This takes a little longer. Instead, your movements are becoming more coordinated. Your body is learning how to move more efficiently and thus can produce more force and speed.

Remember: exercise can be exciting and motivating at first because you see results so quickly. Then as results slow down, exercise becomes monotonous and discouraging. It's important to keep challenging your body and trying new things so you continue to experience improvements.

As you start moving, you realize how great exercise can make you feel when you listen to what your body needs. Sometimes it feels great to push yourself to the limits and step out of your comfort zone. Other times, if you've been stressed at work or feel run down, pushing yourself to the limits can actually leave you feeling more tired and create adrenal fatigue. On these days, a yoga class or an evening walk might be a better choice and leave you more energized.

Remember: there is no right or wrong. You have to listen to your body and do what feels the best. If you are waking up everyday dreading your daily exercise routine, you need to try something different. I'm not saying that exercise is always fun. Exercise can be hard work but it can also be energizing.

Another objective of creating a daily exercise routine is to raise your baseline. You want to raise your perception of what feels difficult. If the most difficult thing you do in your day is carrying the groceries up the stairs to the kitchen from the car, then that activity feels difficult because it's the hardest thing you do every day. If the most difficult thing you do is climb to the top of Mt. Olympus carrying a 20-pound backpack, then carrying your groceries up the stairs becomes easy. You can enjoy your activities of daily living because they become fun and easy rather than challenging and exhausting.

My last point in this segment is the principle of specificity. The type of exercise you choose to do must align with your goals. If you have a goal to run a 10K, you have to run. If you would like to complete a triathlon, you have to swim, bike, and run. You will not become a better runner by riding your bike. If you are feeling stressed out and as if you are running on all cylinders all day every day, your best choice of exercise might not be a strenuous run or high intensity exercise. You might be better off trying a yoga or Pilates class where you can slow you mind and give your adrenal glands a chance to catch up.

When you exercise is also very individualized. We each have a natural biorhythm that is unique to us. Our system fluctuates in highs and lows throughout the day. You might find that you have the most energy early in the morning or maybe it's later at night. You might prefer to exercise first thing so that it's out of the way and you don't have to worry about it all day. Or maybe it's easiest to exercise early so you only have to shower once or maybe that's when your kids are still sleeping and you can sneak out. Maybe you find that evenings are best. It gives you a chance to unwind and process all of your activities from the day. It allows you to slow your brain so you can sleep better. Or maybe the opposite is true and you get a burst of energy if you exercise too late and have a difficult time falling asleep and experience a disrupted sleep pattern. You might find that right after work or on your lunch break is best. We all have other responsibilities and other variables we have to take into account.

Where do you like to be? Do you love being in nature to enjoy the freedom of the great outdoors? You might feel stifled in the gym or be concerned about the germs and recycled air. You might not like the smells or sounds. You might love the feeling you get outside and don't mind braving the elements. Or maybe you live in a climate that is conducive to being outside. Maybe you prefer the structure and consistency a gym brings. You know what you will find inside. You don't have to worry about the weather or if it's still dark at 7am. Perhaps you enjoy the atmosphere and the variety of classes that many gyms offer. Again, there is no right answer. We all have our unique preferences. You might even fluctuate throughout the year, heading to the gym in the winter months and outdoors in the spring and fall and maybe inside in the summer when it's too hot. There is no best choice.

Why do you exercise? This may be obvious but until you really understand why, you will not be consistent in forming a daily habit of exercise. Until you feel it for yourself and appreciate how great movement and exercise can make you feel, you will not be consistent. Do you view exercise as something that you have to do because that's what someone told you, or what you heard on the news, or because that's what "healthy" people do? Does it feel like a chore? Like something else that you have to do each day when you already feel overwhelmed by your to-do list? Wouldn't it be great to exercise because you love it and it is something to look forward rather than something you dread? Sometimes it's just a matter of perspective. Think of the following two statements:

"I exercise because I have to. I read in a book that in order to lose the extra forty pounds that I've been carrying I have to do thirty minutes of high intensity cardio six days per week and strength train three days."

OR

"I exercise because I love the way it makes me feel. I go to the gym daily because I leave feeling more energized and ready to face my day. I do cardio to get my heart pumping and blood flowing. It makes me feel alive. I love seeing the gains in strength that I've made since beginning my exercise routine."

Which person do you think is going to reach their health goals? More likely the second. She has a clear view of why she exercises and is exercising because it makes her feel better and not because someone has told her to exercise.

The media gives such a wide variety of recommendations. How do you know what is really right? The reality is that you have to do what works best for you and your life. You have to be willing to experiment and step out of your comfort zone. You have to make a conscious decision that you want a better life and you are ready and willing to do what it takes. You have to be committed to go for it and figure out what you like and what makes your body feel best. You have to listen to your body, mind, and soul and make decisions confidently knowing that you know your body better than anyone. You are your own best guide. Go for it!

2. Schedule it – Add it into your daily routine

Find time everyday to do something physically active. Even if it's a fifteen minute walk on your lunch break, a bike ride after school with your kids, ten minutes of stretching, abdominal exercises, and push-ups as you are watching TV in the evening. You can schedule larger blocks for a class at the gym or a hike with your dog, or a long bike ride on a sunny day. Just get moving and make it a priority to do something every day.

Exercise becomes easier when it is a habit. You wake up knowing that it is just a matter of deciding what you are going to do, rather than if you are going to exercise. It will become something that you look forward to doing because it makes you feel good. It is not easy. It may never be easy but it will be worth it in the long run.

Keep it simple. Schedule five exercise sessions for the upcoming week. Pick a day and time that work. Pick one or two activities that you want to do and will be consistent with. Then do it!! Stick to your plan and be consistent. Once you have created the routine of exercise, you can experiment with changing the type of activity, duration, and/or intensity to see what makes you feel the best.

3. Hold yourself accountable

You know what exercise you need to do for your body to feel amazing and why you will benefit from a regular exercise routine. You have made a plan and scheduled exercise. Now you have to create a system to hold yourself accountable. To what do you respond best? Are you more successful when you report to someone else? Do you feel proud and accomplished by crossing things off your list or as completed tasks on your calendar? Does having an end goal, like a race to train for or an objective measurement, inspire you? Making a goal for the number of workouts to complete each week may help keep you on track. Making your successes and failures visual will help as well. Write it down.

4. Correlate your behaviors and outcomes

As you try new forms of exercise, make note of how you feel before, during, and after. All forms of exercise have different affects on your mind, body, and soul. Going through the motions and exercising just because you are supposed to will not allow you to achieve the results you desire. The way you feel after a given exercise is sometimes more important than how you feel during. This is the reward you are after: the high that comes from an endorphin release and from accomplishing something you set out to do.

As you shift the perspective of exercise to something you get to do each day, you will embrace it. You will begin to enjoy your life and daily activities to a greater degree. You will see and feel the benefits of daily exercise.

I hope this gives you a different perspective on exercise. How you move or what you choose to do or how long you exercise should not be the emphasis; what's most important is that you get moving. It doesn't have to be all or nothing. Just do something. Movement strengthens your mind, body, and soul. Movement heals.

Action steps:

- ∾ **Decide what you are going to do for exercise this week;**
- ∾ **Schedule it;**
- ∾ **Listen to your body and embrace it.**

Grains

Since early civilization, whole grains have been a central element in the human diet. Common whole grains include brown rice, oats, oatmeal, and buckwheat. Other whole grains are amaranth, barley, bulgur, cornmeal, couscous, kamut, millet, rye berries, spelt, wheat berries, and wild rice. These grains are becoming more available at your local grocery store.

Whole grains provide an excellent source of nutrition. They contain essential enzymes, iron, dietary fiber, vitamin E and B-complex vitamins. Whole grains are an easy addition to your nutrition. They are easy to cook - usually just boiling water. They store well. Grains may be soaked for 1 - 8 hours prior to eating to soften, improve digestibility, and eliminate phytic acid. Phytic acid is a substance that reduces our absorption of minerals such as calcium, iron, zinc, and magnesium and contributes to tooth decay.

Brown rice

Brown rice has all of its bran layers intact, unlike white rice. The bran layers serve to protect the grain and maintain its naturally present nutrients. Brown rice contains the highest amount of B vitamins of all the grains. It also contains vitamin E, iron, amino acids, and linoleic acid. High in fiber and low in sodium, brown rice is composed of 80% carbohydrates. Brown rice promotes good digestion, quenches thirst, balances blood sugar, and controls mood swings.

Prepare brown rice by placing rinsed rice and water into a pot in a 1:2 ratio. For example, one cup rice with two cups water. Bring the water to a boil, and then reduce heat. Cover and simmer for forty-five minutes. You will want to check it at thirty minutes to make sure it doesn't burn. Then, remove from heat and let stand for ten minutes. Fluff with fork and serve. Rice is great with and as leftovers. Make extra and save for another meal.

Quinoa

Quinoa (pronounced KEEN-wah) has been grown and consumed for about 8,000 years. It comes from the high plains of the Andes Mountains in South America. Quinoa has the highest nutritional profile of all the grains. Quinoa is gluten-free and easy to digest. It has high protein content equal to milk and contains all eight amino acids to make it a complete protein. Quinoa is an ideal food for endurance. Quinoa strengthens the kidneys, heart, and lungs. It is high in B vitamins, iron, zinc, potassium, calcium, and vitamin E.

Quinoa is best rinsed with water prior to cooking to remove the toxic bitter coating. Quinoa is prepared similar to rice. Rinse and combine quinoa and water in a 1:2 ratio in a saucepan. Bring to a boil, then reduce heat and simmer covered for fifteen minutes. Unlike rice, quinoa cooks in only fifteen minutes making for a quick weeknight meal. Make extra and serve quinoa for breakfast with nut milk and cinnamon and nuts or add it to your salad for lunch.

Millet

Millet is another great option for use in cereal, soups, and dense breads. A very small round grain, millet is a delicious, wheat-free substitution for couscous. Millet is high in protein, fiber, iron, magnesium, and potassium. Millet is an anti-fungal and reduces candida symptoms. Millet improves breath, supports the kidneys and stomach, and is great for indigestion and morning sickness.

Millet is usually found in the bulk section of health food stores. Rinse millet before cooking and cook similar to brown rice and quinoa. It usually cooks in thirty minutes.

This gives you a brief overview of the benefits of grains. In transitioning to a whole foods diet, grains are an excellent source of nutrition.

Action step:

    ⋘   **Pick one new grain and add it to a meal this week.**

Self Care

Self-care should be second nature to us. If you aren't healthy and functioning at your best, you cannot take care of anyone else. Life is more enjoyable when you take care of yourself. When your mind, body, and soul are in rhythm, you function at a high level. You must put your needs first. These include nourishing your body, getting enough sleep, feeding your soul, being active, and whatever it takes for you to feel great. We each have a baseline that we have to achieve to be able to function and live happy and healthy lives.

We live in a fast paced world. Chores and responsibilities weigh us down. We focus on the details of daily life that we need to accomplish. When prioritizing, we put ourselves last. We take care of ourselves with whatever time is leftover. There is never time leftover. So our needs are never met. To live a fulfilling and happy life you have to put your needs first. This attitude is not selfish. You simply cannot feel guilty about putting your needs before those of your children or your career. You are not taking anything away from anyone else when you take time from your day to exercise or attend to your own desires.

Write out your top ten excuses why you don't put yourself first:

❧

❧

❧

❧

❧

❧

❧

❧

❧

❧

Review your list. Decide which, if any, of these excuses hold merit. Most of them do not. Put yourself first, it is selfish not to.

When you don't put your needs first, you feel unfulfilled. You lack energy and passion to live your life. Ironically, you feel guilty for putting your needs first and guilty for not taking care of yourself. It is time to ditch the guilt.

When you take care of yourself, you give yourself the opportunity to do everything else better. Without opportunity, you set yourself up to fail. Choosing to not take care of yourself is a selfish act. You cannot put your best self out there for your career, your family, and your friends if you do not take care of yourself. By not being your best self you sell everyone short.

I tell my kids, "Mommy is going for a run." They used to whine and cry when I left. I would feel guilty for leaving them but I would tell them, "I run so that I can be a better mommy." After years of telling them this, there is no more whining when I leave. They know it is true. I am a better mommy when I exercise. When I take care of myself, through exercise, nutrition, meditation, or journaling, I am more patient. I am more loving. I am more energetic. I am more organized. I am more productive. I am more giving. I am happier.

Self-care can come in many forms. The obvious forms are physical: eating well, exercising, taking care of our bodies, and avoiding toxins. Self-care also comes in the form of nourishing the mind and soul. We improve our mind through meditation. Turning off our thoughts is an incredibly beneficial practice. Meditation helps to decrease stress, enhance mental clarity, help respiration, reduce chronic pain, and improve sleep. Meditation comes in many forms including breathing, prayer/chanting, ritual/exercise, and viewing art or listening to music. The key to meditation is consistency. Pick a time and place and stick to it.

Stimulate your mind throughout your life. With every new activity learned, new synapses in the brain are formed. A synapse is the structure that permits the neuron to pass an electrical signal to another cell. Your brain is composed of millions of synapses to transfer signals. As movements are repeated, those synapses become stronger and other synapses fall away. Infants have billions of neurons in their brain. As they learn new skills, new synapses are formed and that area of the motor cortex becomes more developed. Over time these areas are reinforced and become larger and other areas that aren't used as much go away. Every time you learn a new skill you expand your motor cortex. A study showed that individuals who continually learned new activities and stimulated their brain in new ways were more likely to have a full recovery following a stroke. Choose a new skill to challenge yourself mentally and physically.

When you feel at your best, what is happening around you? What are the key pieces in your puzzle that have to be intact for you to be your best?

We all have requirements in our life that we must do daily, weekly, monthly, and yearly to function and to live the life we desire. What do you need to do to take care of yourself to be happy and healthy? These are not things you know you should do or the things that you are supposed to do. These are the basic requirements you have to be happy and healthy. These requirements are highly individualized. They may include going to a yoga class, drinking water, journaling, socializing with friends, intimacy, being in nature, eating fruits and veggies, drinking your daily green smoothie, massage, socializing with friends, etc.

You may know exactly what I'm talking about and have a great understanding of what makes you tick. But, if you are in a place in your life where you are feeling stressed, unhappy, overwhelmed, or unfulfilled, you may have a harder time pinpointing these self-care minimums. Refer to the "Self Care Minimum Exercise" in the Intuitive Health Workbook to help you pinpoint your minimum requirements.

Self-Care Minimums

Read each question then spend two minutes writing. Do not stop writing for the entire two minutes. Leave the judgment behind and fill in the blanks. List whatever comes to mind.

Without _____ I lose myself.

When I feel most connected to my center I am _____.

When I feel most connected to something larger than myself I am _____.

I can live without _____ but not for long.

Review your lists. Highlight the items that are repeated. These are your self-care minimums. These are the things that make you who you are and make you happy. Focus on these items to create a life that you love. Make these minimums a priority and incorporate them into your daily routines.

When you take care of yourself, you do everything else better.

Action steps:
- Determine your self-care minimums;
- Make time every day this week for one act of self-care.

Protein

Protein is made up of amino acids, which are the basic building blocks for the human body. The body makes many amino acids; however, the body cannot make essential amino acids. Essential amino acids must come from food. Protein is crucial for vital functions, regulation, and maintenance of the body.

How much protein and what types of protein we should consume are among the most debated nutrition topics. Some argue that large amounts of high quality lean animal meat are necessary for optimal health. Others advocate for a plant-based diet. Experiment with what works for you and your body. There is no magic number for the amount of protein to be consumed daily. Listen to your body and give it the fuel it needs.

Some signs of too little protein consumption are: sugar and sweet cravings, feeling spacey and jittery, fatigued or weak, experiencing unintended weight loss, anemia, loss of healthy color in facial area, and change in hair color and texture. In some extreme cases skin inflammation and a potbelly may occur. Note that very few Americans are protein deficient.

Some signs of too much protein include: low energy, constipation, dehydration, lethargy, heavy feeling, gaining weight, sweet cravings, and feeling tight or experiencing stiff joints. With excessive protein, the body becomes overly acidic and enters a state of ketosis. The kidneys become taxed due to excess pressure to filter toxins and waste. Foul body odor, halitosis, and calcium loss occur to compensate for the acidic state of the body.

Protein sources can be divided into animal and vegan sources. Choosing animal or vegan sources is a personal decision.

Examples of animal protein sources:
Meat - common sources are chicken, turkey, beef, lamb, buffalo, duck, ostrich, and game.
Egg - quick and inexpensive. Eat the entire egg to receive the total energy.
Fish - contains healthy omega-3's. Note some fish, including mackerel, swordfish, tilefish, and shark, contain high levels of mercury and should be consumed in moderation.
Dairy - yogurt, butter, ghee, buttermilk, and milk (cow's, goat's or sheep's).

Many people have negative reactions to cow's milk. Buy organic to avoid growth hormones and antibiotics.

Examples of vegan protein sources:

Grains – whole grains including quinoa, rice, millet, buckwheat, and oats.

Beans – smaller beans such as split peas, mung, and adzuki are easier to digest. Soaking beans overnight also improves the digestion.

Nuts – usually considered a fat but peanuts have more protein than most other nuts.

Leafy greens – broccoli, spinach, kale, collard greens, bok choy, romaine lettuce, and watercress all contain protein. They also are major sources of magnesium, iron, and calcium.

Seeds - chia, flax, hemp, pumpkin, sesame, and sunflower are high in nutrients and provide anti-inflammatory and cardio vascular benefits. They also contain vitamin E, fiber, and omega-3's.

Protein powder – look for high quality ingredients as many are highly processed. May use in addition to whole natural foods but not recommended in large quantities.

Protein bars – some are healthier than others based on ingredients and the amount of processing. Many contain refined carbohydrates, sugar, chemicals, highly processed protein isolates, and artificial sweeteners. Should not be meal replacements.

Soy – edamame (baby soybeans), tofu (soybean curd), and fermented soybeans (tempeh, miso, and tamari). Soybeans are the most difficult beans to digest. May not be great to consume highly processed soy such as soymilk, soy meat, and soy ice cream. Soy is one of the most genetically engineered crops, so buy organic whenever possible.

Soy milk – highly processed and fortified with nutrients

There are many choices when it comes to protein. As with all foods, listen to your body. Choose the type of protein that makes you feel best. Look for the signs of too much or too little protein and make adjustments.

Action steps:
- ✎ **Experiment with eating protein this week and note how you feel;**
- ✎ **Try a new form of protein.**

Posture

Improving your posture can have a profound impact on your daily life. Our self-awareness, self-confidence, and mood are reflected in the way we carry ourselves and vice versa. The energy we release and the way others view us directly correlate with our posture. When we engage with someone who is full of life and energy, their energy is contagious. When someone smiles or laughs, it is human nature to smile or laugh with them. When someone stands up tall and carries an aura of confidence, it is human nature to replicate that behavior. When you enter a room where people are down and discouraged, you can feel it and see it in those people immediately.

There are numerous benefits gained both internally and externally when you improve your posture. According to Wolf's Law, bone grows and remodels based on the forces that are applied to it. In other words, our bone structure is constantly changing. Muscles are attached to bone through tendons. Every time a muscle contracts, that muscle applies a force to bone, which causes the bone to grow or remodel its structure. This is why weight-bearing activity is so beneficial in maintaining bone density. The forces applied by our muscles continually contracting stimulate bone growth. Over time, our bone structure changes. Our posture has a direct affect on how our bones remodel.

Posture can be defined as structural or functional. In structural posture, the bones have been remodeled to a specific shape, which affects the range of motion of a joint. Conversely, functional posture is dictated by muscle activity and has more flexibility for movement. For instance, we often see people with a hunched-forward posture. The thoracic spine (the area of the spine that is attached to the ribs) is forward flexed, or kyphotic. If the posture can be reversed and the person can extend the upper back or at least stand up tall, this posture is functional. If the curve is unable to be reversed, it is structural. The bones have remodeled in such a pattern that the muscles can no longer alter the position. This occurs when the bones lack bone density and the strength to withstand the forces of gravity. This is an extreme example but in my work as a physical therapist, I address poor posture in every patient.

Another example is how posture affects the position of the head and neck. Many people suffer from chronic headaches. In our society, more and more people have jobs that require prolonged hours sitting in front of a computer. We sit down and begin working without considering how we sit in our chair or how our desk is arranged. Over time, our shoulders hunch. Our head draws forward. We slouch in our chair. Not only does this put a lot of strain on our neck and the base of our skull, which can lead to headaches, but it is also a low energy position. Conversely, sitting up tall while working at your computer improves focus, increases productivity, decreases back pain and headaches, improves breathing by allowing your ribcage to expand, and raises your vibration (an emotional feeling that is sensed instinctively). Improving your posture affects all those around you as well. When you sit up tall, others will follow.

To understand what makes good posture, you need to understand some basic anatomy of the spine. The pelvis is connected to the sacrum, which is connected to the lumbar, then thoracic, then cervical spine, with the occiput and head resting on the top. The spine is shaped like an 'S' with an additional curve.

The lumbar spine is curved to the front of the body, called a lordosis. The thoracic spine curves to the back of the body, called a kyphosis. The cervical spine, or neck, is curved to the front again. We naturally position our spine so that our eyes are on the horizontal to improve our visual field. Thus, the position of the pelvis affects the entire chain. If the pelvis tilts forward, the lumbar increases the size of its curve and the thoracic and cervical spine adjust so our eyes remain level. If the pelvis tilts backwards, our spine rounds and we increase the curve in our neck and our head comes forward so that our eyes remain level. The goal is to achieve a mild curve, which varies in size with every individual, throughout the spine. This begins with positioning the pelvis in neutral.

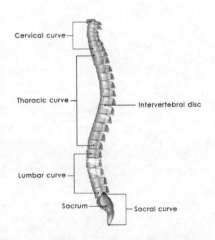

Finding a neutral pelvis position:

Picture your pelvis as a bucket. Put your middle fingers on the prominent bones on the front of your hips and wrap your thumbs around to the back of your pelvis. Now, rock your pelvis forward and backwards. Imagine there is water in your 'bucket' and when you tip your pelvis forward, the water will spill out the front. When you tip it backwards, the water will spill out the back. Shift your pelvis so that it's level so no water will spill out. This is your neutral pelvis position.

Achieving good sitting posture:

First, look at the relation of your hips and knees. Your hips should be slightly higher than your knees with your feet firmly planted on the floor. This position puts your pelvis in a neutral position thus improving the alignment of the rest of your spine. Second, the shoulders should be resting comfortably away from your head and slightly drawn back. If you pull them too far back, it will cause your ribcage to flare open and put strain on your lower

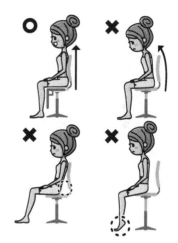

back. Third, your head should be resting directly on top of your spine. Adjust your seat height and/or computer screen height so it's at eye level so that your head remains in neutral.

Feel the benefits of this posture. The challenge is that it takes strength to maintain this posture. Use your chair to your advantage and sit back so that your pelvis is supported in this position. Use a towel roll or a small pillow if needed to support your spine. This way you are 'resting' in a position of good posture.

Another place to apply good sitting posture is in your car. We spend many hours every week driving. Poor sitting habits develop because of the position of your car seats. In newer cars, there are many adjustments that can be made to improve your posture. Use them to your advantage and apply the above principles. Tilt the seat upwards to raise your hips slightly above your knees. This may also mean bringing the seat slightly closer to the steering wheel so you can reach the gas pedal and brake. Use the lumbar support to support your spine and pelvis. Adjust the height of your steering wheel so your shoulders remain relaxed away from your head and slightly drawn back. Adjust your rearview mirror so your head is in neutral (not looking up or down) when viewing.

Stand tall:

As you make these changes in your posture, feel how it affects your mood and overall well-being. Feeling down in the dumps? Try changing your posture. When we feel down, we naturally slouch, our head and shoulders move forward and our weight is transferred to our heels. Instead, stand up tall. Shift your

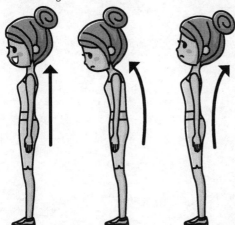

weight to the balls of your feet and lightly squeeze your inner thighs together. Feel the difference. This subtle shift raises your energy and vibration. Your head is now in alignment with your spine, you are in a position to attract and give off energy. Feel your spirits lift.

The way you hold yourself and your mannerisms have a huge impact on the way others perceive you. When you feel shy or vulnerable, you naturally raise a hand to your throat or in front of your mouth. Feeling threatened - you cross your arms and close yourself off. Feeling confident - you stand tall and proud. Feeling playful - you are light on your feet and your eyes are bright. Your posture tells a lot about you.

How do you want the world to see you? Feeling good about yourself is contagious. Share the love.

Action steps:

- ∾ **Make adjustments to your sitting posture at your desk and in your car;**

- ∾ **Feel the difference your posture makes on your mood and energy.**

Fats

There are many different types of fats, including trans fats, saturated fats, omega-3s, omega-6, Omega-9, polyunsaturated fats, and monounsaturated fats. Much conflicting information surrounds which are healthy and which are not. It is confusing to know which fats we want to incorporate in our diet and which we should avoid.

Fats are important in your diet because they supply essential fatty acids, which are required for good health. The source of fats remains controversial and recommendations have changed over the years. Fats provide energy for low intensity activity.

Monounsaturated Fats

Monounsaturated fats generally are considered heart healthy and should be eaten daily. They are found in avocados, olives, olive oil, nuts, sunflower oil, seeds, halibut, and mackerel. They are liquid at room temperature and become solid when chilled. They raise good HDL and lower bad LDLs, which are forms of cholesterol.

Polyunsaturated Fats

Polyunsaturated fats are also considered heart healthy in moderation. They are found in salmon, sardines, mackerel, herring, trout, fresh tuna, flax seed, walnuts, flax seed oil, and soybean oil. They are liquid at room temperature and when chilled. These are the omega fats, including omega-3, omega-6, and omega 9. Strive to eat cold-water fish three times per week and plant-based polyunsaturated fats often.

Saturated Fats

The consumption of saturated fats remains controversial. Saturated fats are solid at room temperature. They are found in beef, poultry, pork, cow's milk, coconut, avocado, palm oil, and full-fat dairy. It is generally recommended to consume saturated fats in moderation because they can potentially increase risk of heart disease.

Trans fats

Trans fats may be found in margarine, processed foods, candy, chips, soda, flaky pastries, and some peanut butters. They raise LDL (bad cholesterol) and lower HDL (good cholesterol). This leads to plaque buildup in arteries and increases the risk of heart disease. Trans fats should be avoided entirely. Avoid products with partially hydrogenated oils on the ingredient label.

Action step:

৶   **Read labels and eliminate trans fats from your diet.**

Sleep

Are you getting enough sleep? The amount of sleep required is highly individualized but the recommendations for an average night's sleep are eight hours per night. If you are not sleeping enough, you are depriving your body of its chance to thrive. These are the primary benefits of sleep.

Repair and rejuvenate. The body regenerates while you sleep by producing protein molecules, which build new cells and repair the damaged ones. The major restorative functions, such as muscle growth, tissue repair, protein synthesis, and growth occur primarily at night. Sleep improves your immune system, which allows you to fight off infection.

Brain plasticity. Sleep plays a critical role in brain development in infants and children. The quality and quantity of sleep impacts learning and memory in adults as well. How this occurs is still unclear but it is suspected that the neural connections that strengthen our memory are forming during sleep. Just one night of sleep deprivation has shown a decrease in brain tissue.

Weight control. Short-term sleep deprivation has been linked to feeling hungrier, eating larger portions, and preferring high calorie and high carbohydrate foods. Chronic sleep deprivation is linked to an increased obesity risk.

Improved health. First and foremost, you just feel better when you sleep. Chronic sleep deprivation increases your risk of heart disease, hypertension, diabetes, colorectal and breast cancer, stroke, and obesity. In addition, chronic sleep deprivation decreases sperm count and increases your mortality rate.

When it comes to sleep it is not only quantity but also the quality of sleep that counts. Sleep can be disrupted by numerous factors including: caffeine, stress, sugar, late night eating, using electronic devices, watching TV, and exercise. If you are struggling to get a good night's rest here are some ideas that might help.

- Avoid caffeine close to bedtime;
- Take a warm bath with lavender or Epsom salts;
- Turn off all electronic devices one hour prior to bedtime;
- Listen to quiet and relaxing music;
- Meditate or read a book;
- Make sure your room is dark and cool (64 degrees is ideal);
- Eat dinner at least two hours prior to bedtime;
- Avoid sugar before bed. Eating sugar to close to bed time will cause hypoglycemia and wake you up;
- Exercise at least three hours prior to bedtime to allow your cortisol levels to drop. Cortisol is a stress hormone that will keep you alert that increases with exercise;
- Make it a priority to get enough quality sleep. Plan ahead and go to bed.

Sleep is important. Whatever is preventing you from going to bed can wait until the morning. With eight hours of rest, you will be more productive and have more energy to accomplish all that you need to the following day.

Action step:

- **Make it a priority to get eight hours of sleep every night this week.**

Portion Control

Portion sizes continue to grow. The portions we eat today are much larger than what they were twenty years ago. Since we are all different sizes, the best method for measuring portions is to use your own hand. I weigh less and my hands are smaller than my husband's, thus it would make sense that my portions are smaller than his as well. I apply this model to my children as well. They are much smaller than me. They are too frequently served portions that are much too large for them.

General rule of thumb:

Rice, pasta, fruit, veggies – size of your fist;

Meat, fish, poultry – size of your palm;

Nuts, raisins – amount you can hold in your hand without it overflowing;

Chips, popcorn, pretzels – amount you can hold in both hands together;

Peanut butter and hard cheese – size of your thumb;

Cooking oil, butter, mayonnaise, sugar – size of the tip of your thumb.

Action step:

∽ **Be conscious of your portions this week and apply these guidelines.**

Healthy Snacking

We put a much greater emphasis on meal planning and preparation for dinners than for breakfast, lunch, and especially snacks. Snacks are fillers between meals and are frequently eaten on the go. We get in the habit of grabbing something quick from the pantry to provide a quick burst of energy. These pantry snacks are loaded with sugar and preservatives and provide little nutrition. Snacking can be a great way to provide your body with extra nutrients to get through the day. With a little planning and prep work, whole food snacks can be just as quick and convenient as the pantry snacks.

3 Keys to Healthy Snacks

- **Keep it real;**
- **Make it available;**
- **Add fat and protein;**
- **Have a backup plan.**

1. Keep it real

Whole food is always better than processed. It contains vital minerals and nutrients that your body needs. The more nutritious the snack, the longer you will feel satisfied and full and refrain from continued grazing. Our typical snack food - such as crackers or granola bars - lacks nutrients and is made with fillers, high fructose corn syrup, and partially hydrogenated oils (trans fats). Unless the crackers are organic, they will contain hybridized wheat, which contains more gluten and has been manufactured to be addictive. Once you start eating these crackers, it's hard to stop.

The same is true with processed snacks that are high in sugar. Fruit snacks and fruit rollups, which are frequently a go to snack for kids, are loaded with sugar and do not contain fruit. They raise blood sugar, creating a high to make you feel good. The pancreas releases insulin to lower the blood sugar. The blood sugar dips below normal causing a crash. You then crave more sugar to raise your energy and mood again. Fresh fruit contains natural sugar and fiber so blood sugar remains more stable. Fresh fruit is a much better choice.

Dried, or dehydrated, fruit can be a great option for on the go. Read the ingredient label. The only ingredient should be fruit. Be cautious of added sugar.

2. Make it available

The appeal of snacks in the pantry is their convenience. They are always ready to be thrown in a bag or given to a hungry child. Whole food can be just as convenient with a little planning.

At dinner, slice up extra vegetables, such as bell peppers, zucchini, mushrooms, and carrots. Store them in airtight glass containers for easy snacking. These are also great additions for lunches.

Some fruit - apples and pears - can be washed ahead of time. Cut up watermelon and store it in the refrigerator for a convenient snack. Berries should only be washed right before eating.

Make snack bags of nuts and dried fruit. Nuts are a great on the go option. Replace your candy dishes with dishes full of nuts. Because nuts are high in fat (the good kind) and calorie dense, it's difficult to overindulge. You will feel full and satisfied.

Make peanut butter balls and store them in your freezer for an easy on the go snack (1 C natural peanut butter, 1 C oats, and ¼ C honey. Mix together, roll into balls, and freeze.)

3. Add fat and protein

Add healthy fats and protein to your snacks to make you feel full and satisfied. It takes longer for your body to break down fats and protein than simple carbohydrates.

Healthy fats are found in avocado, nuts, oils (coconut and olive oil are my favorites) and whole dairy products. Make guacamole to dip veggies, add avocado to a salad or sandwich. Saturated fats have received a bad rap for causing heart disease but new studies show no correlation. Dairy products made with whole milk are less processed and will make you feel more satisfied. They are also a more complete source of protein than the fat free versions.

We most often think of animal sources when we think of protein, such as meat, fish, eggs, and dairy. There are also a handful of vegan protein sources as well. Protein is found in whole grains (rice, millet, quinoa, buckwheat, and oats), beans, nuts, seeds, and leafy greens (broccoli, spinach, kale, collard greens, bok choy, watercress, and romaine lettuce).

With such variety you can get creative with your healthy snack combinations.

4. Backup plan

This is all great when things go well. But what happens when you have sick kids or life gets crazy and you haven't made it to the grocery store. Let's face it, it's hard to plan ahead and always have healthy snack options available. It's a necessity, especially with young kids, to have a backup plan. Having healthy options in the pantry can be a lifesaver. When choosing pantry food, I encourage you to **read the ingredients**. You will be amazed how much snack food still contains high fructose corn syrup, partially hydrogenated oils, and artificial coloring. These are the big three to avoid. The amount of calories or percentage of fat is not as important. Look for whole food ingredients and minimize added sugar. Sugar should not be one of the first three ingredients. The fewer ingredients, the better.

Action step:

<ul>
<li>∾ Replace one unhealthy snack with a healthy snack of your choice each day this week.</li>
</ul>

Controversial foods

My primary emphasis is on adding in whole foods and changing habits to improve your health. I am an optimist. I focus on the good things rather than dwelling on the bad, especially when it comes to food. I encourage my clients to celebrate all of the good food they eat and focus on how it makes them feel. They want more of that feeling so they are encouraged to make better choices. However, this book would not be complete without a discussion about controversial foods. The primary topics in our world today are avoiding genetically modified organisms (GMOs), gluten, added sugar, trans fats, and artificial dyes.

Genetically modified organisms

Genetically modified organisms (GMOs) are plants or animals that have been genetically modified with DNA from bacteria, viruses, or other plants and animals. GMOs has been engineered to withstand the application of an herbicide or to provide an insecticide. Biotech industries suggest that they also withstand drought, increase yield, and enhance nutrition. These benefits have not been proven to be true. What we do know is that most countries including Australia, Japan, and the European Union, do not consider GMOs safe and have banned them for consumption. The United States government has approved GMOs. In the U.S., GMOs are in as much as 80% of conventional processed food. The most common GMOs are soy, cotton, canola, corn, sugar beets, Hawaiian papaya, alfalfa, and squash (zucchini and yellow).

The long-term health effects of GMOs remain unclear. Some studies have linked GMOs to decreased fertility, lowered immunity, organ damage, accelerated aging, and possibly an increase in allergies, particularly soy allergies. GMOs make it possible for allergens in one food type to emerge in a completely different species. GMOs can contaminate existing species being grown organically. GMOs are found to transfer genetically modified DNA into the DNA of bacteria living in the human stomach.

Unfortunately, we won't know whether GMOs are really safe for years to come. Purchasing organic food is a good option to reduce exposure; however, these crops may still be contaminated. Look for the Non-GMO Project label.

Decrease your consumption of processed foods with hidden ingredients, primarily soy, canola, and corn.

Gluten

Gluten is the protein found in wheat. Over time wheat has been hybridized to increase the amount of gluten to make bread with a more appealing texture. Hybridization involves crossing different strains of wheat to generate different characteristics. Some breeders have even used chemicals to mutate the wheat. Hybridized wheat contains 28 chromosomes, rather than the 14 chromosomes found in your great-grandmother's wheat. This causes the body to produce antibodies to fight inflammation. The result is celiac disease, gluten intolerance, cancer, irritable bowel disease, depression, and many autoimmune diseases. According to Dr. Mark Hyman, M.D., the other problem is that hybridized wheat, even whole "grain," also contains a starch that causes you to gain weight and a chemical drug to make you crave more.

Should everyone avoid gluten? The answer is you should avoid gluten if you have celiac disease or gluten sensitivity. Otherwise gluten is not bad for you. The excessive amount of gluten found in hybridized wheat is what is causing gut inflammation. It is wise to avoid all hybridized wheat products. Avoid foods with "whole grain" wheat, "wheat flour," and "white flour" on the ingredient label. Look for "whole wheat flour" on the ingredient label and buy certified organic grains.

Added sugar

The refinement of sugar from sugar cane was invented in India in the fourth century. It was considered a very potent drug and used sparingly. Christopher Columbus carried sugar with him on his second voyage to the New World. In the 1600s, sugar was exported to Europe, where only apothecaries handled it. It was extremely expensive. It became quickly apparent that sugar was highly addictive and the demand for sugar became high. In the 18th century, the Caribbean became the world's largest source of sugar. They could supply sugar cane using slave labor. The heightened demand and production of sugar was driven by a change in the diets of many Europeans. They began eating jams, candy, tea, chocolate, and other processed foods.

As the use of sugar increased, conditions of malnutrition and toxicity became prevalent. Heart disease was not documented until the 1930s. Over time, health deteriorated as sugar consumption increased. In the 1950s, high-fructose corn syrup was developed and by the 1970s high-fructose corn syrup replaced sugar in soft drinks and most processed foods. The use of high-fructose corn syrup has been linked to numerous diseases such as metabolic disease, diabetes, heart disease, and obesity.

In 2012, the World Health Organization made the recommendation to cut all sweetened foods to below 10% of calories. For a 2200 calorie/day diet, this means limiting total sugar intake to 220 calories per day, or 57 grams. One gram of sugar contains 3.87 calories. This includes natural sugar, or sugar naturally found in whole foods such as fruit. The consumption of naturally occurring sugar is not as detrimental because it is combined with fiber. Natural sugar does not have the same impact on your health because of how it is processed by your body. This is the equivalent of one king size Snicker bar or one Cinnabon cinnamon roll. The American Heart Association recommends limiting added sugar to twenty three grams for women and thirty eight grams per day for men. We have an epidemic; our young children are suffering from adult diseases, including diabetes and heart disease. These are primarily caused by our excessive sugar intake. The average intake of sugar in the Standard American Diet (SAD) is around 459 calories per day, or 119 grams of sugar. This is more than double the recommendation.

Refined sugar is four times more addictive than cocaine. It's no wonder that we all consume more sugar than is recommended. To classify a substance as addictive, the following behaviors occur when consumed:

1. Loss of control – it is difficult to stop eating sugar once you start;
2. You continue to use it even though you are clearly aware of its health consequences;
3. Withdrawal symptoms – headache, general malaise when you remove sugar;
4. Relapse – Americans relapse rate on sugar is 97%;
5. Progressive and terminal – you need more and crave more over time;
6. Deadly – heart disease, diabetes, and cancer.

Refined sugar is manufactured for addictiveness. It is a white powder. It is not food. It is a high calorie drug. When you ingest sugar, your insulin levels rise, which raises serotonin levels. This is very similar to heroine. It affects the opiate receptors in the brain in the same way. The rise in glucose levels makes us feel good. Then glucose levels taper and we want to feel good again so we consume more sugar. Sugar substitutes are also highly addictive.

The other problem is that sugar is rarely consumed on its own. We most frequently ingest sugar in other foods. We combine sugar with wheat and starch, such as in cookies, cakes, breads, muffins, etc. As previously discussed, hybridized wheat contains excessive amounts of gluten. The more gluten, the more addictive it is. Chocolate contains caffeine in addition to sugar, which also contributes to addictiveness. Casein, found in dairy products, has the same addictive affect on the brain as well.

High fructose corn syrup (HFCS) is a cheap sweetener made from corn. It was introduced into our foods in the 1970s as a cheaper sweetener than cane sugar because of the government farm bill subsidies. This allowed for the average size soda to go from 8oz to 20oz with little financial cost. The support for HFCS is that it is that same as sugar and it should be good for you because it is made from corn. But, HFCS is highly processed and not a naturally occurring substance.

HFCS is primarily found in processed foods; including NutraGrain bars, Pop Tarts, Ritz crackers; condiments including ketchup, barbeque sauce, and salad dressing; candy such as Skittles, Lifesavers, and bars; and in sweetened beverages such as lemonade, Capri suns, soda pop, and sports drinks. HFCS is also found in bread, cookies, cereals, and yogurt. HFCS is found in children's pain relievers and fever reducers. Read ingredient labels and you will be surprised at how frequently you find HFCS. Companies are making an effort to remove HFCS from their products; however, the replacement ingredients are still not whole foods. Companies continue to add more and more chemicals to our food.

Cane sugar (sucrose) consists of glucose and fructose in a 50-50 ratio. For sucrose to be digested, enzymes must first break fit down into glucose and fructose. Fructose is sweeter than glucose. HFCS also consists of glucose and fructose but in a 55-45 fructose to glucose ratio and an unbound form. No digestion is required so glucose and fructose more rapidly enter your blood stream. HFCS does not stimulate insulin or leptin production so appetite suppression from the brain does not occur. Thus, HFCS contributes to overeating and excessive calorie intake, especially in the form of sweetened beverages.

If the blood sugar is not immediately used up in some form of exercise, it is converted into fat and stored in the body as excess weight. Fructose goes right to the liver and triggers lipogenesis, which is the production of fats like triglycerides and cholesterol. This causes fatty liver disease, which affects 70 million Americans.

Even when used in moderation, HFCS is a major cause of heart disease, obesity, cancer, dementia, liver failure, and tooth decay, according to Dr. Mark Hyman.

I believe that our best choices for food come in their whole form. When we eat the way nature intended, we are most healthy. The obesity rate in adults has doubled and the obesity rate in children has nearly tripled from 1970 to 2013. It is hard to dispute the correlation between the rise of obesity and the introduction of high fructose corn syrup in the 1970s.

There is a large genetic component to addiction, as taught in Alcoholics Anonymous. Since sugar appears to have the same affect on the opiate receptors in the brain, if you are addicted to sugar, you have to eliminate it and treat it an addiction. Our ability to manage sugar intake is highly individualized. One person may be able to eat sugar in moderation, while for another they experience a loss of control. Sugar that is found naturally in foods, such as fruit, does not have the same effect on the brain because these foods contain fiber. One thing is clear, we would all benefit from minimizing our consumption of added sugar.

Trans fats

Manufactures create trans fats through a process called hydrogenation, which turns liquid oils into solid fats. Trans fats lengthen the shelf life of processed foods and improve the taste and texture. They can be found in margarine, crackers, cereals, cookies, granola bars, candies, baked goods, chips, salad dressing, fried foods, and many more processed foods.

Trans fats raise LDL "bad" cholesterol and lower HDL "good" cholesterol. The LDLs clog arteries causing heart disease. HDLs help to clear the LDLs from your arteries. Trans fats contribute to heart disease and diabetes. Trans fats should be avoided; however, this requires reading the ingredient labels closely. If a product contains partially hydrogenated oils, these are trans fats. In the United States, a product that contains less than 0.5 grams trans fats is labeled as containing 0 grams of trans fats. In order to avoid trans fats, you must read the ingredients.

Artificial dyes

Artificial dyes are chemicals that are added to processed foods to enhance colors, add color to colorless food, and provide consistency to foods where there is a variation in color. Artificial coloring has been approved by the FDA and is frequently used in processed foods in the United Sates. However, it remains unclear if these artificial dyes are really safe. The British government and the European Union have taken steps to eliminate the use of artificial coloring in foods. They use natural coloring instead. Artificial coloring has been linked to hyperactivity in children, cancer (in animals), and allergic reactions. Some examples that are most commonly found in processed food are Yellow 5, Red 40, and Blue 2.

Artificial dyes are still considered safe by the FDA; however, the FDA has acknowledged that Red 4 is a carcinogen, which is a substance or agent that is directly involved in causing cancer. Red 40, Yellow 5, and Yellow 6 are contaminated with known carcinogens. Some artificial dyes are made from chemicals derived from petroleum, a crude oil.

Adding artificial coloring to foods is designed to make processed foods more appealing to children. Artificial dyes are added to candy, baked goods, macaroni and cheese, fruit snacks, and beverages. It is disconcerting that children consume the most of these potentially dangerous chemicals.

I read labels and avoid ingredients such as Red 40, Red 3, Yellow 5, Yellow 6, Blue 1, Blue 2, and Green 3.

This discussion of controversial foods is included to educate you so you can make the best decisions for you and your family. These are purely my opinion and my thoughts. As with everything in life, you need to make decisions that are best for you. The more you know, the more empowered you become to make you own informed decisions.

Detoxify Your Home

Our environment plays a huge role in our health. Our immune system faces a constant assault by chemicals and free radicals that cause degenerative disease. These chemicals come from cleaning products, furniture and textiles, and paint and decorations. You can make a profound improvement in your health by reducing your exposure to these toxic chemicals.

Cleaning supplies

Toxic chemicals are present in generic cleaning products. These chemicals are often unregulated and many products do not list their ingredients. The chemicals we use to clean our home are frequently inhaled, absorbed into our body through our skin, or ingested through indirect contact. Have you ever washed your kitchen counter with a chemical cleaner and then eaten food off the counter? When choosing cleaning products, it is best to look for 5 ingredients or less and primarily plant-based. You can also choose to make your own cleaning products with baking soda, vinegar, or lemon. I use Norwex cleaning cloths and only use water to clean and sanitize my entire home. To learn more about Norwex, visit alligardner.com/products.

Furniture and textiles

Manufacturers add flame-retardants to mattresses and children's clothing to comply with fire regulations. The chemicals used in these retardants are known to cause poor brain development, as well as learning, behavior, and memory problems in children. Adults (18 years old and older) spend one third of our life in our beds and children (ages 3-17 years old) spend more than half of their lives sleeping. On average, infants and toddlers sleep between 11 and 19 hours every day. Invest in a mattress and sleepwear made of natural materials, such as untreated cotton and wool.

Many chemicals are found in carpets and furniture as well. Stain resistant treatments, antimicrobial properties, and antistatic agents are all toxic. Use natural materials whenever possible. Choose hardwood floors if you are moving to another home or renovating.

Ideas to improve your home environment

As with nutrition, it can be overwhelming to overhaul your environment all at once. Begin by implementing one small change at a time.

- Replace generic cleaning supplies with natural alternatives; Grow plants indoors and open windows to allow fresh air and sunshine to filter rooms;

- Consider purchasing air filters for bedrooms and workout areas;

- Use glassware instead of plastic for food storage whenever possible;

- Never put plastic in the microwave;

- Replace old plastic water bottles regularly. Over time the plastic breaks down and releases chemicals into your beverage;

- Compost kitchen scraps;

- Recycle trash and buy recycled goods;

- Switch to energy saving light bulbs and use appliances efficiently;

- Avoid toxic chemicals on your lawn and flower beds.

Section VI

Enjoy Your Life

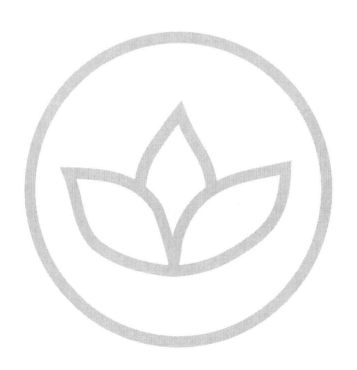

Live, Laugh, Learn, and Love

Live

The final step in improving your health is living your life. Great health is not a destination. It is a journey. That means there is no end. You have met your goals and improved your health, now you maintain and enjoy it. Great health empowers you to live out your dreams. When you are healthy you can reach for the stars. Dream big. Live the life you want. This four-step process is designed to put you in control of your life, your health, and the decisions you make. As you figure out what works best for you, your body, and your life, you don't have to work as hard. It becomes a habit. There will always be challenges along the way. As long as you remember your why, you will stay on track. That track won't always be a straight line, but you will continue to move in the right direction. As you become healthy, you focus on living and enjoying your life.

Laugh

Enjoy the journey. Take time to look at the big picture. We get so caught up in the details of life that we forget our purpose. As a mom, I get hung up on laundry, picking up toys, cooking meals, and cleaning. I forget to laugh and enjoy the best parts of being a parent. The smiles and giggles and new outlook on life are the highlights that kids bring. With health, it is easy to get so wrapped up in what you are supposed to eat, counting calories, and restricting meals. It's easy to forget the big picture. Health is not about counting calories and eating the right things. Health is a vehicle to live the life of your dreams. When you envision your life and your life purpose, counting calories is probably not on your list.

In the Franklin Covey training, participants experience the Big Rocks experiment. Imagine two large buckets, one is empty and the other is half full of small pebbles. The small pebbles represent the details of life. Next to the buckets are 10 large rocks representing the big picture: family, career, exercise, health, home, vacations, etc. When the big rocks are placed on top of the small pebbles, they do not all fit in the bucket. However, when the big rocks are placed in the empty bucket they all fit. As the small pebbles are added to the bucket, they fill in the empty spaces between big rocks. Everything fits. Instead of focusing on the details of life, focus on the things that are most important. The big rocks bring you joy, happiness, fulfillment, laughter, and a sense of purpose. The small pebbles keep life moving forward.

Learn

There is always more to learn. The more you learn, the more empowered you become. As you learn more, you gain the ability to form your own opinion and trust your opinion instead of relying on those of others. There is an abundance of information. You decide what feels good and what is relevant and leave the rest. As you learn more and experiment, you become more empowered to manage your own health and well-being. I enjoy learning about what works for others: what they believe and what they are doing. It doesn't mean that I have to replicate that in my own life. Years ago, as I sought my path, I attended lectures, read blogs, and felt so inadequate. Why couldn't I gulp down super greens everyday like my friend? Why couldn't I eat a diet of primarily raw food like David Wolfe? I realized that if I bought every supplement recommended, I could spend millions. I tried many supplements. Often I never felt a difference. Do I really have to take fish oil because Dr. Oz recommends it? What about the opinions that most fish oil contains high levels of mercury and is toxic? As I learned more, I gained confidence to listen to my body and do what works best for me. Most of all, I've learned not to judge or criticize. We each have to do what works best for us. I am no longer critical of myself. I no longer feel like I am not healthy enough or fit enough or happy enough. I am living the life of my dreams. I am incredibly grateful.

Love

Being healthy and eating well generate a mindset. Make the decision that you love yourself. Decide that you love your family enough to make changes. Decide that improving your health is more important than the two minutes of satisfaction the donut in your office break room will give you. It is not about sacrificing or giving up anything. It is about loving yourself. It is about giving you life. Make health a priority and a non-negotiable. Without health, everything else in your life suffers.

I love my life. I love the woman I am and the woman I continue to become. I love sharing my knowledge with you. Love yourself. Love the journey you are on.

This Is Not the End.
It Is the Beginning.

The best things in life are worth working for. Changing your habits and improving your health are not easy. You have given yourself the best gift. You have decided to take the first steps to improving your health and your life. As you have worked through this book, you have learned that by incorporating one new health habit at a time, it is possible to make big changes. I have attempted to give you all of the information you need to begin your journey. Sometimes that is enough to get the ball rolling in the right direction. Sometimes, though, it is not enough. You need support, personal guidance, and someone to be accountable. I have created a variety of programs at *www.alligardner.com*, to further help you to achieve your goals.

You are most likely to have success when you have support with changes in your nutrition and lifestyle. This support can come from a loved one, a friend, a coach, or a mentor. Find someone with whom you can be yourself to share your struggles and successes. Once you start opening up, you will find that you have the answers. You sometimes need someone else to open your eyes to the answers. You also learn that we all have struggles and fears that are holding us back from becoming our best selves. Once you move past these fears, there are no boundaries to your potential. Ask for help. Receive help. We are programmed to believe that giving is more important than receiving, that it is a sign of weakness to receive help. It is a sign that you are unable to do it yourself. Let go of this belief. There is an equal, energetic exchange that accompanies giving and receiving. In order to give, someone or something has to be on the other end to receive. When you receive help, you are allowing someone to give you assistance. You will find yourself on both ends of the spectrum. Embrace it. Receive help when it is given to you.

My intention has been to empower you to find your own path: to let go of the shoulds and coulds and ifs; to let go of the excuses that have prevented you from becoming your best self. You are amazing. You are improving your life one step at a time. You are creating an environment and a lifestyle that foster health. By surrounding yourself with whole foods, you make it easier to make great decisions. By surrounding yourself with people who support you and your journey, you make it easier to stay true to you and to stay on track to reach your goals.

People who live the longest have established habits that make health part of their daily life. They don't think about it or stress about it. It just happens. They get enough sleep. They have a great support and social network. They eat whole foods that nourish their body. They are active and exercise regularly. They attend religious services or embrace their spirituality. They create a home environment that promotes happiness and life. They have a strong sense of value and purpose. They enjoy their life and live it to its fullest. Of course they go through the highs and lows along the way but overall they have created habits that enable health and life.

There is always a next step. There is always another goal to achieve. When you feel like your progress has stalled, review the goals you set a few months ago. Celebrate how far you have come. Keep your vision in mind and create a life that will bring it to fruition. Anything is possible. I wish you a lifetime of health and happiness.

Appendix

Worksheets

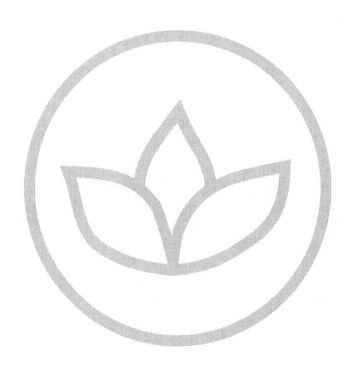

Why Health?

What does it mean to be healthy to you?

Why Health?

Do you meet your own definition of health?   ○ Yes   ○ No

Why or Why not?

How will you feel when you are healthy?

How will you look when you are healthy?

How will being healthy affect your life?

How will being healthy affect those closest to you?

What do you feel is holding you back from being healthy?

How long have you been working to improve your health?

What has prevented you from improving your health?

Why do you want to improve your health?

Are you ready and willing to do whatever it takes to improve your health?

Who Are You?

What was your childhood like? Describe your family and home life.

What did you do for fun? What activities?

What foods did you eat?

Were your parents or caregivers healthy? O Yes   O No

Were they active? O Yes   O No

How did your parents or caregivers handle stress?

Did they exercise, turn to food, drink alcohol or smoke, yell?

Do you see any of these behaviors in your own life? If so, which ones?

How do you handle stress? How does it affect your life?

Does this bring up any behaviors that you would like to change?

If so, what are they?

Why do you want to change these behaviors?

How do these behaviors relate to your health?

Fears/Support Worksheet

How will your life improve when you achieve your goals?

Who will be affected by your achievement?

How will you feel if you don't achieve your goals?

How will those closest to you be affected if you don't achieve your goals?

What fears do you have around achieving your goals?

How will you overcome those fears?

What support do you need to achieve your goals?

Who will support you?

Why will you benefit from this support?

When will you ask for support?

Where will you receive support?

Limiting Belief Exercise

Write out fifteen beliefs that you have about nutrition, exercise, and health. Examples: "No pain. No gain." This is not true. You do not have to hurt to benefit from exercise. Healthy food tastes bad. Not true. You just haven't found what you like. Overtime your taste buds adjust as your eat whole, unprocessed foods. You body will crave what it needs. Exercise is boring. You haven't found that type you enjoy or you're ready for something new.

- ∽
- ∽
- ∽
- ∽
- ∽
- ∽
- ∽
- ∽
- ∽
- ∽
- ∽
- ∽
- ∽
- ∽
- ∽

Write down where you heard each belief. Is it something from your childhood or something you read or heard or something you know from experience?

Put and X through the beliefs that you know are not true.

Circle the beliefs that you question.

I encourage you to explore these beliefs.

Re-write a new list of YOUR beliefs about health, food, and exercise.

15 NEW Beliefs About Nutrition, Exercise, and Health.

    ❧

    ❧

    ❧

    ❧

    ❧

    ❧

    ❧

    ❧

    ❧

    ❧

    ❧

    ❧

    ❧

    ❧

The Circle of Life

Discover which primary foods you are missing, and how to infuse joy and satisfaction into your life.

What does YOUR life look like?

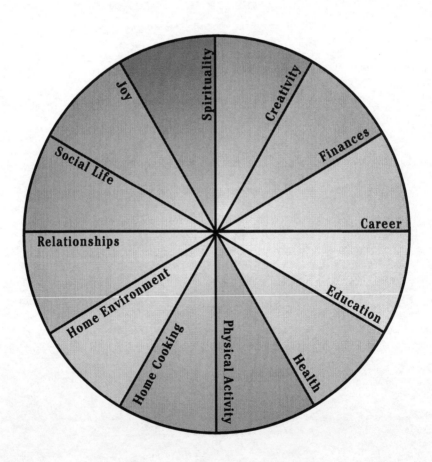

1. Place a dot on the line in each category to indicate your level of satisfaction within each area. Place a dot at the center of the circle to indicate dissatisfaction, or on the periphery to indicate satisfaction. Most people fall somewhere in between.

2. Connect the dots to see your Circle of Life.

3. Identify imbalances. Determine where to spend more time and energy to create balance.

List your top 3 areas that need improvement.

&

&

&

S.M.A.R.T. Goals Worksheet

Specific. Your goals must be specific and clearly defined.

Measurable. Your goals must be measurable.

Achievable. Your goals must be achievable.

Realistic. Your goals must be realistic.

Timely. Your goals must have a time component.

Examples of SMART goals:

"I will eat at least one serving of greens everyday in January."

"I will engage in physical activity for at least thirty minutes, five days each week."

"I will have date night with my significant other every other week."

"I will write in my gratitude journal five times each week"

As you write you goals, make sure to address

Primary and Secondary Foods.

6 Month Goals

- ❧

- ❧

- ❧

Three Month Goals

- ❧

- ❧

- ❧

One Month Goals

- ❧

- ❧

- ❧

Daily Habits Worksheet

Make a list of those things that you do almost every day, i.e. your morning routine.

Which habits are improving your health?

Identify which habits are detrimental to your health.

List three new healthy habits to implement this week.

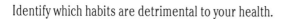

What Is Your Life Purpose?

Create a list of the top five things you value most in life. For instance: time for family, loyalty, honesty, health, integrity, freedom, activity, creating things, teamwork, independence, generosity, security, etc.

≈

≈

≈

≈

≈

Which one do you value most?

≈

≈

≈

What are you great at?

What things do you look forward to doing every day?

Name three things that come naturally and easily to you.

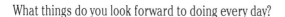

If you could do anything, be anything, what would it be?

Create a life purpose statement that sums up who you are and what you are meant to be.

Write down this statement and place it somewhere you can read it everyday.

Vision Exercise

Write out a detailed ten-year vision. Where do you see yourself in ten years? What is your ideal life? What if you have all of the resources, time, money, and support you need. What do you truly desire?

Next, keeping your ten-year vision in mind, **write out your three-year vision.** What things must happen in three years for you to be on track to reach your ten-year vision?

What do you need to achieve in the next year to be on track to achieve your three year and ten year visions?

Set 3 SMART Goals for **the next year**.

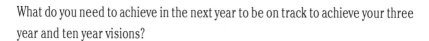

Write down your goals and place them somewhere you can read them everyday."

My Nutrition Blueprint

A nutrition blueprint is a set of guidelines that you follow as you make food choices. It is not meant to be a set of hard and fast rules that you follow to a T. Make a list of guidelines you can strive for in making nutrition decisions.

∽

∽

∽

∽

∽

∽

∽

∽

❧.

❧

❧

❧

❧

❧

**Over time your blueprint will change
as you learn more and your body
adapts to eating healthy foods.**

Self-Care Minimums

Read each question then spend two minutes writing. Do not stop writing for the entire two minutes. Leave the judgment behind and fill in the blanks. List whatever comes to mind.

Without _____ I lose myself.

When I feel most connected to my center I am _____.

When I feel most connected to something larger than myself
I am _____ .

I can live without _____ but not for long.

Review your lists. Highlight the items that are repeated. These are your self-care minimums. These are the things that make you who you are and make you happy. Focus on these items to create a life that you love. Make these minimums a priority and incorporate them into your daily routines.

When you take care of yourself, you do everything else better.

Appendix

Examples

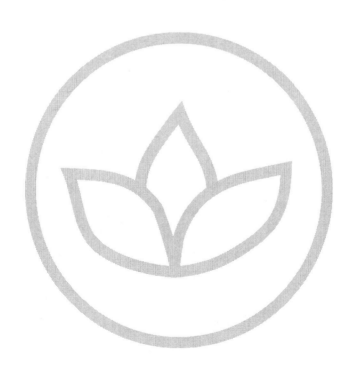

Example One

Susan was in her mid 30s. She wanted to lose weight and improve her energy. She came to me expecting a meal plan, an exercise plan, and accountability. As we began, it became apparent that she was extremely unhappy with her career. Each time we talked, the discussion gravitated toward her job and the stress and unhappiness it created. She was using food to cope with the stress her job created. The more stressed she felt, the more she ate comfort foods. The more sugar she ate, the less energy she had and the less she exercised. The less she exercised the more she ate because she felt bad about herself. This self-perpetuating cycle continued.

We began by adding in greens to her diet every day. She experimented with a green smoothie and having a green salad for lunch. She realized it took planning to get to the grocery store every weekend to prepare her meals for the week. As she integrated the habit of going to the grocery store, she began to buy nuts and fruits and veggies to cut up for snacks. It worked best for her to divide up her foods into snacks size baggies for the week. Every time she hungered for a snack, she had something prepared. We addressed adding in healthy fats to fuel her body, such as nuts, avocados, and healthy oils (coconut and olive oil). She drank more water and reduced her alcohol intake. She introduced different grains and proteins to her meal plans. She began to love the process of grocery shopping and cooking at home. We incorporated education about each new food group and ways to incorporate them every other week at our session.

In the meantime, she focused on creating a vision for her career and to figure out how to live her passion. As she created a plan to change jobs, her stress reduced, and her moodiness lifted. She was concerned about not exercising consistently and skipping a lot of workouts. I emphasized that she needed to figure out what she loved to do and find something she could be excited about doing. She had completed some triathlons but really despised running. She loved lifting weights and working with her personal trainer. She committed to exercise five days a week.

Halfway through our program, she identified exercise as her keystone habit. She realized that when she began her day with exercise, she ate better, she handled stress at work better, and she slept better. She was encouraged to integrate exercise into her daily routine. It became something she looked forward to and could not live without.

She quit her job to follow her passion in a new career. She became excited to go to work and new opportunities began to present themselves. She was happy and felt like she had created new lifelong habits. She planned out her meals for the week, grocery shopping to keep healthy, whole food options available at home. She was amazed that her unhappiness in her career could have such a profound influence on her health. She left my program a different person than when she began. I was honored to be part of her remarkable transformation. She did the work and she was committed to forging a new path.

Example Two

Judy came to work with me to improve her energy and her overall health. She was a stay at home mom of three young kids and struggled to manage her life. She felt low on energy and complained of frequent headaches. She craved sweets almost every night. She wasn't as concerned about her weight but wanted ideas to improve her diet and her family's. She felt unprepared at mealtime and it became a frantic rush to put food on the table. She frequently skipped breakfast and her snacks were the convenience foods she fed her children, primarily goldfish crackers and fruit snacks.

We began by introducing a daily habit of eating greens. She loved the idea of the green smoothie, but wasn't so sure about putting spinach in a smoothie. She began with more frozen berries and less spinach. It was quick and easy to prepare and she could drink it on the go. She also found that she could make an extra large smoothie in the morning and have it for an afternoon snack. After the second month, she was using more greens and less fruit. She also noticed that her headaches were not as frequent and she didn't crave sweets as frequently in the evening.

When she completed the circle of life exercise, she realized that the areas of most dissatisfaction were physical activity, health, and social life. She recognized that she took care of her family and friends, her household duties, her volunteer obligations first. Her needs always came last. She took care of herself with whatever time was leftover at the end of the day. There was never any time leftover. She identified three habits to take care of herself. First, she would exercise every morning before her children awakened. Even if it was only fifteen minutes, it still counted. Second, she scheduled time every week to connect with friends. Often it was a play date with a friend and her children, but she also incorporated evening gatherings with her husband and friends. Finally, she would eat three meals everyday and replace the goldfish crackers with fruit and veggies.

The first couple of months were difficult. She was too tired to get up early to exercise. She beat herself up for her laziness. The meals required more planning and organization than she realized. She created a meal plan for the entire month for dinner. Meals repeated themselves but they were family favorites so it worked. She identified three lunches that she enjoyed and rotated through those. If she kept it simple, it worked. She really enjoyed the time spent with friends. She realized that it energized her and made her happier at home.

After four months, she was experiencing steady energy throughout the day and feeling better. She continued to struggle with exercise. She experimented with exercise in the morning and in the evening. Ultimately, she decided that she needed to go to bed earlier and get up in the morning. She recruited help from her family to clean up the house in the evening and she was able to go to bed earlier. She was then able to get up and exercise, which made her whole day feel less rushed. Her keystone habit was an early bedtime.

At the conclusion of our six months, Judy had met her goals of improving her energy and providing consistently nutritious meals for her family. She learned that when she took care of herself first, she could take care of everything else better. She slowly added in one behavior at a time and over time she made huge progress. It was wonderful to experience her success.

My Nutrition Journey

I am healthy and happy. But, I am in no way perfect. I strive to live my life in balance and moderation. I am not always successful; nonetheless, that is my goal. I always strive to improve my health and that of my children. Achieving health is a constant evolution. The challenge is that life is always changing. Just when I think I've got it, something shifts and I start the process again. Each time the process seems to get a little easier. Some things have become a habit, like my daily green smoothie. Other things continue to be a challenge for me, like meal planning. I'm always working on something.

Growing up, my focus was more on athletics than food. I never thought much about what I put in my body. I ate frozen waffles for breakfast, peanut butter and jelly sandwiches on white bread or bagels with cream cheese for lunch and home cooked meals or Domino's pizza for dinner. I'm sure I had some fruits and veggies. Salad was definitely not a staple.

In college, I focused on playing basketball, classes and studies, and my social life. Again, good nutrition was not something I gave much thought to. I ate what was around and convenient, probably not many fruits and veggies in the school cafeteria. Even after graduating from college as I began my triathlon obsession, I didn't focus on the quality of food I ate. I started to think more about what I was eating but I had very little whole food in my diet. I was newly married. We both worked full-time jobs. We ate at restaurants or ordered take out frequently. I ate foods that I thought I was supposed to eat, especially as an athlete. I didn't give much thought to what I felt best with. I was never a great meat eater so I substituted with a lot of dairy and whey protein powder in my mid-20s. After years of cereal and cow's milk followed by a vanilla latte on my way to work did I finally realize that my stomach hurt every day. I guess I just thought that's what happened when you ate. At that point, I had my first revelation that I should not be drinking cow's milk. Once I stopped, my stomach issues began to improve. I did continue to force myself to eat a lot of protein, mostly chicken. I was under the impression that as an endurance athlete I had to eat 1.2 g of protein per kilogram body weight, which meant about 90 g of protein every day. That was a lot for me. I read books about nutrition for endurance athletes and tried to follow the guidelines.

After the birth of my first baby when I was 30, I was introduced to protein smoothies. I dropped my baby weight very quickly. I was nursing and had only gained about 25 pounds during my pregnancy. Before long, I actually weighed less than my pre-pregnancy weight. I looked great but I felt awful. I learned that it's not just about what you weigh on the scale. I was exhausted and incredibly moody. I soon realized that I very rarely ate anything before noon. I obsessed about running and getting back in shape. I focused on caring for my newborn. My needs always came second. A friend recommended protein smoothies. I believe my original recipe was 10 ounces water, one banana, 1 cup frozen berries, one scoop of whey protein isolate powder, 1/2 cup oatmeal and 1/2 cup yogurt. It was a meal and I knew I was headed in the right direction. I was still fairly gassy and bloated but my energy improved significantly. I felt a desire to return to everything I did prior to my pregnancy, including triathlons. I became more consistent in my diet and exercise although it was a juggling act with my little one. I focused on feeding my baby healthy foods, primarily vegetables and fruits. She ate well while I continued to guzzle pizza. Because I exercised, I believed that I could eat whatever I wanted. At this point, I opened my own Pilates studio. Folks frequently asked questions about nutrition and I gave my opinion freely. I didn't have much else to offer other than my opinion so I began reading everything I could find to become an expert. I took a few nutrition courses and sought out guidance from three different nutritionists. Each gave me different advice; none of which fit with my life or the foods that I enjoyed. One person told me I was allergic to almost everything including dairy, wheat, onions, garlic, melons, and nuts. This really limited my diet and was not sustainable. Another recommended that I eat 90 grams of protein everyday and weigh all of my food. He wanted me to eat a turkey sandwich with eight ounces of turkey. I gagged it down for a couple of weeks before I realized it was not for me. Another recommend about $150 monthly in supplements that I needed to take every day, including multivitamins, fish oil, calcium, vitamin D, glutamine, and a variety of other things I can't remember. He also wanted me to eat all whole foods. It was overwhelming. He was telling me to go from A to Z when I was only ready to go to B. My diet improved. I changed the ingredients and portions in my daily protein smoothie. I ate more fruits and veggies. I was still eating a lot of meat protein. Around this time, I was introduced to the green smoothie girl. That was eye opening for me. I began putting spinach into my smoothie. I loved it. The more I read, the more I believed that good nutrition was the key to health.

When my second baby was born, she was extremely colicky. She cried and cried and I always felt like something I was eating made her cry. I had her tested for food allergies. The tests always came back negative. I thought that when I ate ice cream and a lot of dairy she cried more. My pediatrician did not support my theory because the tests always came back negative. Because I was training for another Ironman, I resisted giving up dairy. I needed to get my 90 grams of protein in everyday and eating a lot of dairy made that possible. My little girl had four ear infections and had tubes put in her ears before her first birthday. I blamed it on the daycare she attended.

Then I began experiencing difficulty swallowing. A doctor diagnosed me with eosinophilic esophagitis. Following an endoscopy, I was told this was an allergy to something I was eating but I just needed to take medication for reflux and a steroid forever. The doctor told me my symptoms would be tolerable and manageable as long as I took the medication. I was disappointed in our healthcare system. It was my first experience with a doctor pushing medication on me rather than finding the cause of the problem and making changes to fix it. I sought alternatives including acupuncture, dousing, and a lot of supplements. I consulted with a naturopathic doctor; yet, I was still not in control of my own health. I yearned for the knowledge to put me in charge. I read everything I could find on nutrition. It was confusing yet fascinating at the same time. Everyone had a different opinion on what to do, what not to do, what to eat, what not to eat, best times for eating, not eating at certain times. My head spun with information.

My baby was diagnosed with pneumonia when she was 15 months old. She spent two nights in the hospital. She came home from the hospital with a nebulizer, with an inhaled steroid to be given daily and whenever she started getting snotty. I still believed she was intolerant to dairy but where would she get her calcium and vitamin D if I didn't feed her cow's milk? She was supposed to drink cow's milk when she turned one, right? I followed the advice of my pediatrician and continued to feed her whole cow's milk.

The following spring, I enrolled in the Institute of Integrated Nutrition (IIN). I wanted to study nutrition from a holistic view, to learn how to improve the health of my family and myself. I hungered for more knowledge about nutrition so I could make informed decisions to improve our health. It was an amazing journey. I learned about so many different dietary theories. One theory argued that dairy could be highly mucus producing in some people. We eliminated dairy from my daughter's diet and there was an instant improvement in her health. I was amazed that a change in nutrition could have such a dramatic effect. I learned about so many different theories. Each seemed very logical. The most important thing I learned is that everyone has different nutrition requirements. The only way to figure out what works best for you is to try different things. Nutrition is like a giant experiment.

I sought guidance from a naturopathic doctor for my baby as well as myself. The naturopath tested us for food intolerances with the ELISA test. The test showed that my daughter was primarily sensitive to wheat and dairy. For me the list was extensive and also included wheat and dairy. We eliminated wheat and dairy for six months. It was not easy. Our symptoms improved and he opened my eyes to a new path of health. I learned that our primary immunity comes from the gut. Without a healthy and balanced digestive system, our immune function is diminished. Our environment and the toxins we are exposed to daily affect our health and immunity as well.

A year later, I learned about the healing power of essential oils. We have incorporated a daily practice of doTERRA essential oils. I have been able to avoid Tylenol for headaches and ibuprofen for muscle aches and joint pain by using peppermint and lavender instead. This is a new journey and one that I am thoroughly enjoying.

I believe that our nutrition as a family continues to improve. We are striving to teach our kids the importance of good nutrition and good choices. I never imagined that I would have kids that asked for chicken nuggets from Wendy's. That's hard to admit, after all, I am a health coach. It's not a regular meal but like sweets I believe moderation is key. I still drink my green smoothie everyday. I have also incorporated doTerra essential oils into my daily routines. To learn more about doTerra essential oils please visit www.alligardner.com/products.

I have a new green smoothie recipe.

Green Smoothie Recipe

2 cups Water

3 cups of greens

1 banana

1-2 cups frozen berries

1 Apple

1/2 scoop of Green Smoothie Girl plant-based protein powder

2 drops of ginger doTERRA essential oil

2 drops of lemon doTERRA essential oil

I love it and most days I add a green salad as well. My diet consists primarily of fruits, vegetables, lean protein, legumes and whole grains. I would love to be more consistent with making homemade baked goods and snacks. My goal is to eat whole foods and make great food choices 90% of the time. That means of the 35 meals I eat a week (3 meals/day plus 2 snacks) I strive for 31 great meals. That gives me four meals a week that I can cut myself some slack. I have the freedom to eat out or make other decisions without beating myself up. For me it comes down to planning. My poor food choices come when I don't plan ahead.

You can see from my journey it's not about being perfect. It's about slowly making changes to improve your health and listening to your body. You just do the best you can do. I don't believe that it has to be all or none. Being healthy is not just about eating the right food; it's also about living a life that works for you.

I hope that you can relate to some of my journey and realize that we are too critical and judge ourselves by what we think we see in others. We beat ourselves up over our poor decisions. Focus on the good things you do for yourself each day. As you continue to add in better habits, you will feel the difference and see the difference and this will be the encouragement that you need to continue. Welcome to your journey.

My Exercise Journey

Let me give you a personal example of how I have moved through a variety of exercise in my life. With my diverse background in athletics, I am willing to engage in just about any type of activity. In my early childhood, I began skiing and swimming competitively. I loved the rush of the wind in my face on the ski slopes and the adrenaline of standing on the starting blocks at the swimming pool waiting for the gun to pop. I played tennis, tried diving, rode bikes, and shot hoops. My parents were active and encouraged us to participate in a variety of activities. It was all I knew. I loved it so I never complained. When I was eight, my younger brother began playing soccer. I showed up to every practice and every game hoping they would need an extra player so I would be able to play. I was the only girl on their team. I loved the team aspect and working with others for a common goal. I began playing soccer on a girl's team the following year. I continued to ski but soon realized that the team sports were calling my name. In high school, I played volleyball, basketball, and soccer. This led to being recruited to play basketball at the University of Puget Sound. I was so excited for the opportunity to play a sport in college. I was obsessed with exercise at this point and remember pushing myself to the limits during wind sprints and then spending time in the gym on the stair stepper. I found my place as a leader on my team. I loved supporting my teammates as they struggled to make the time cut off for the 1.5 mile run. I frequently volunteered to run extra wind sprints to support my teammates. I not only loved how I felt pushing my body but I loved how it felt to support my teammates in accomplishing their goals as well. When I became sick the winter of my senior year, I began to realize that more exercise is not always better. I also realized that to function at my best, exercise played a crucial role in my happiness. Moderation was key.

When I graduated from college, I began the next era of my athletic endeavors: triathlon. I entered my first sprint triathlon and was hooked. I loved training and pushing my body to see how long it could go. I initially began reading everything I could about training for triathlon. I mostly followed training programs from books I read. My brother-in-law encouraged me to sign up for my first Ironman in 2005. Although Ironman is an individual sport, having a partner to train with was crucial. I began to work with my first triathlon coach, Scott Browning. He wrote up programs that, upon first glance, seemed impossible. But, I found I was able to push myself farther than I ever imagined. Three months into my training, I began to realize that qualifying for the Hawaii Ironman was not only possible but also a very realistic goal for me. I was disciplined with my training and focused. Between training, recovering from my training, and working as a Physical Therapist fulltime, I didn't have much time or energy for anything else. My spouse was incredibly supportive but felt left out in the process. I completed my first race with an amazing time of 10 hours and 39 minutes. Unfortunately, I finished fifth and missed qualifying for Hawaii by just over a minute. I was disappointed but determined to qualify. I signed up for the Florida Ironman five months later. This time, I restructured my work schedule and training plan. I was able to create more time with my spouse and thus maintained a better overall balance to my life. I finished in second place and secured a spot in the Hawaii Ironman the following year. Ironically, my time was 1 minute faster. During my training, I developed an overuse injury in my left knee. I took some time off and tried to rehabilitate it but without success. I had knee surgery and began the process to come back for the Hawaii Ironman 9 months later.

Having knee surgery was actually a great learning experience for me. I realized that I was treating my patients the way I was taught in Physical Therapy school. My approach was very cookie cutter and not individualized to my patients. I tried following my programs to rehabilitate my own knee but instead found myself creating a new path, one that was very specific to me. It changed the way I worked with my patients for the better. I began to see each of them as individuals and treated them that way. It is interesting to me now that I look back that I never sought help or guidance from another Physical Therapist. It was implied by myself and my coworkers that I was a Physical Therapist and should treat myself. In hindsight, I would have benefited from another set of eyes.

I recovered and trained, with the help of Scott, to compete in the Ironman World Championship in Hawaii. During my training, I began incorporating Pilates. I loved it. I loved the way I felt energized after each workout. I left feeling like I had just done something great for my body, like I was building myself up rather than breaking myself down. I was immediately hooked. Competing in the Hawaii

Ironman was one of the most incredible experiences in my life. I crashed on my bike the day before the race, which derailed my game plan. It became all about finishing and achieving my goal. I finished and felt proud and relived that it was over.

I was struggling with the same knee problems, but on my other knee. I had another knee surgery two weeks later. This began a period of contemplation and soul searching. Who was I doing this for and why? It was beyond being fit and healthy. I was intrigued by the idea of becoming a professional triathlete. I was actually totally unbalanced in my life and my relationships suffered. My life had become all about me, and my training. The vast majority of my training was done alone, aside from an occasional masters swim workout or spin class. It was isolating. I was straying from my life purpose and not being true to myself. I was fit but actually carrying 10-15 extra pounds. How is that possible? I was training about 30 hours a week and very conscious of eating everything I was "supposed" to eat. I realized that I was not healthy and had to follow my heart. What I wanted most in life was to be a mom.

Two months later, I became pregnant with my first baby. I walked throughout my entire pregnancy. I loved it. There was no watch on my wrist telling me how long or how far I had gone, only the sounds of my breath and footsteps and those of my dog next to me. We walked through neighborhoods and in the mountains on trails. It was wonderful. I began to realize that I could be fit and healthy without running myself into the ground. I also began the process to become a certified Pilates instructor. I felt so connected to the work and began incorporating Pilates into my Physical Therapy practice. After my baby was born, I jumped right back into training and pushing myself. I would train to the point of burnout and then back down again. I did four triathlons in this period, including a Half Ironman. I was struggling with who I had become as a mom and holding onto who I once was. I was unhappy working in a Physical Therapy clinic. I felt like it was all about how many patients I saw rather than the quality of care I was able to give them. I decided to leave my practice and open a Pilates studio. I was fortunate to have the support of my husband as well and my parents and in-laws to help with our daughter.

Then I got pregnant with my second baby. I felt great and continued running, cycling, and swimming throughout my pregnancy. After my daughter was born, I felt like I had to do another Ironman. I don't know why. What did I have to prove and to whom? I had two children, was running my own Pilates studio, teaching Pilates classes, commuting 45 minutes to work, and my husband was a college basketball coach who was rarely present. I trained for seven months and did the Ironman when she was my second child was fifteen months old. I had a new coach for this race, Cari Junge. She was amazing and a mom so she realized that my training had to be more about quality of my workouts rather than quantity. I felt great and was holding on but one month before the race my infant was hospitalized with pneumonia for two nights. She became my priority and my training suffered. I completed the race but I struggled throughout. I was sleep deprived and not 100% trained. My mind wasn't focused on the race; I was more concerned about what my kids were going to eat than what I was going to eat during the race. It was a bad sign. I suffered through, but finished.

I took some time off to evaluate my relationship with exercise. Why did I need to push myself to such extremes? What was I trying to prove? I had begun experimenting more with my diet and working to create balance in my life. Balance with two kids, a dog, my own business and a husband who was a collegiate basketball coach? That seems like an oxymoron. But, for the first time, I began exercising to improve my energy and lift my spirits. It felt good to give myself time to heal and ponder. Most of my exercise was in the form of walking. We had a new puppy and I loved my morning walks, especially with coffee in hand. I loved the fresh air and peace that I got first thing in the morning as the sun was rising. I often felt guilty, like I still needed to "exercise" later because a walk wasn't really exercise. It was just a walk. I also decided that I had too much going on and was not able to be fully present with my children. I decided to close my Pilates studio and become a stay at home mom. I was so happy and content although I realized how difficult it is being home full time.

Shortly thereafter, my husband decided to change careers and we moved back to our hometown of Salt Lake City. I began teaching Pilates again and became pregnant with my third baby. For the first time in my life, exercise really took a back seat. I fit it in when I could and when I felt up to it. I was exhausted. I had two busy children and was in the midst of a lot of change in my life. I was just hanging on.

Now, as I am settling in to my life, I still make exercise part of my daily life but I have learned to let it go. I use it as a form of self-care, a chance to fill my tank that is frequently running low. Some days, there's time for a run or a bike ride but I can't stress or feel down about what I am not doing. There will come a time in my life that I will have more time and my emphasis will shift again. I still feel more productive and energized when I exercise but the emphasis is definitely on quality and what makes me feel great.

I tell you my story so you can see how I have evolved. Life is dynamic. We are constantly changing and so are our daily needs for food and exercise. There is no one size fits all guide to either. Just when you think you have it all figured out, things change. Life is a work in progress. It's not about the destination, it is the journey that counts. So, put one foot in front of the other and get moving.

Acknowledgements

This book is a culmination of many years of study and focus. I would like to extend loads of thanks to all of the wonderful people who helped me on my journey. Thanks to you and your willingness to share, I have accumulated a wealth of knowledge.

I would like to those who made this book possible. A big thanks Janet Tingwald at Mission Marketing Publishing for believing in me and encouraging me to keep writing. To John Eggan, thank you for sharing your expertise and writing system; it was amazing. I would like to give an enormous thank you to Dr. Tim Morrison for editing my book. You helped me find my voice and create something I am incredibly proud of. To Robyn Openshaw, Amanda Moxley, Matthew Burnett, and Reed Davis thank for your kind words. You each played an instrumental role by entering my life when I needed you most. To Celeste Rockwood-Jones, thank you for your vision in creating alligardner.com and Karen Cleveland for putting it all together. To Kristina Schmidt, thank you for your wonderful designs on my worksheets, cover and book layout. To all of my friends and supporters, thank you for continuing to read my newsletters and encouraging me to complete this book.

Finally, to my family, thank you for your patience and unyielding support. It has been a roller-coaster ride. I greatly appreciate your love and willingness to join me on our journey of health.

For a free download all of the
worksheets found in this book visit
alligardner.com/bookbonus.

Subscribe to my newsletter for
more tips and information about
nutrition and healthy living.

Learn more about
additional products and my
health coaching programs.

Contact me at
alli@alligardner.com.

Thank You!

In health and happiness,

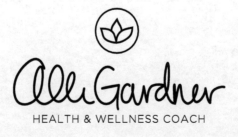

HEALTH & WELLNESS COACH

Made in the USA
Charleston, SC
02 May 2015